# THE *Wellbeing* Bible

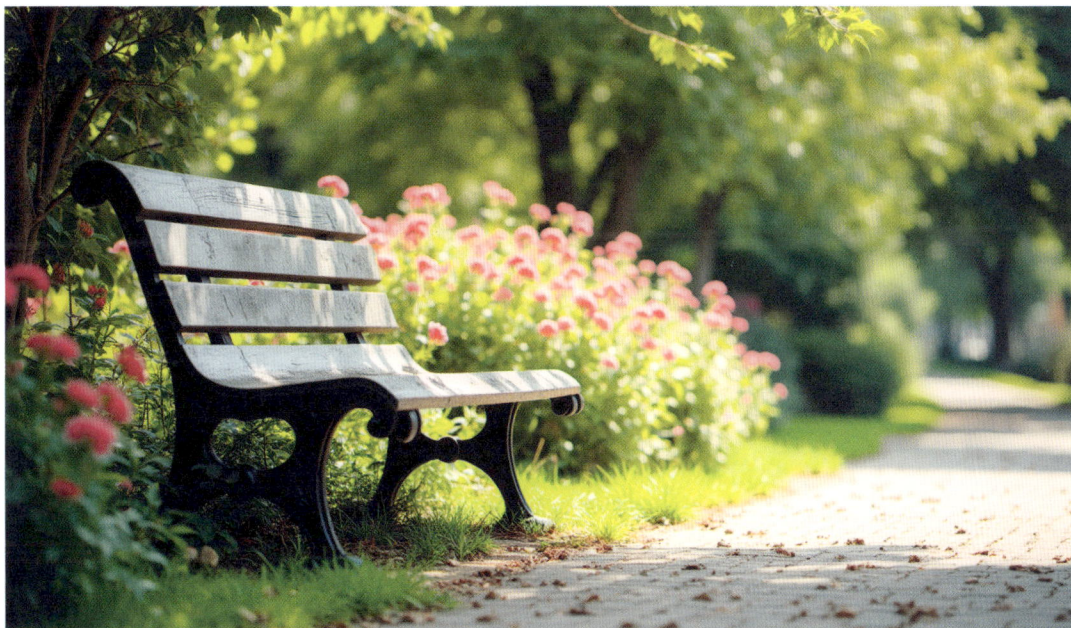

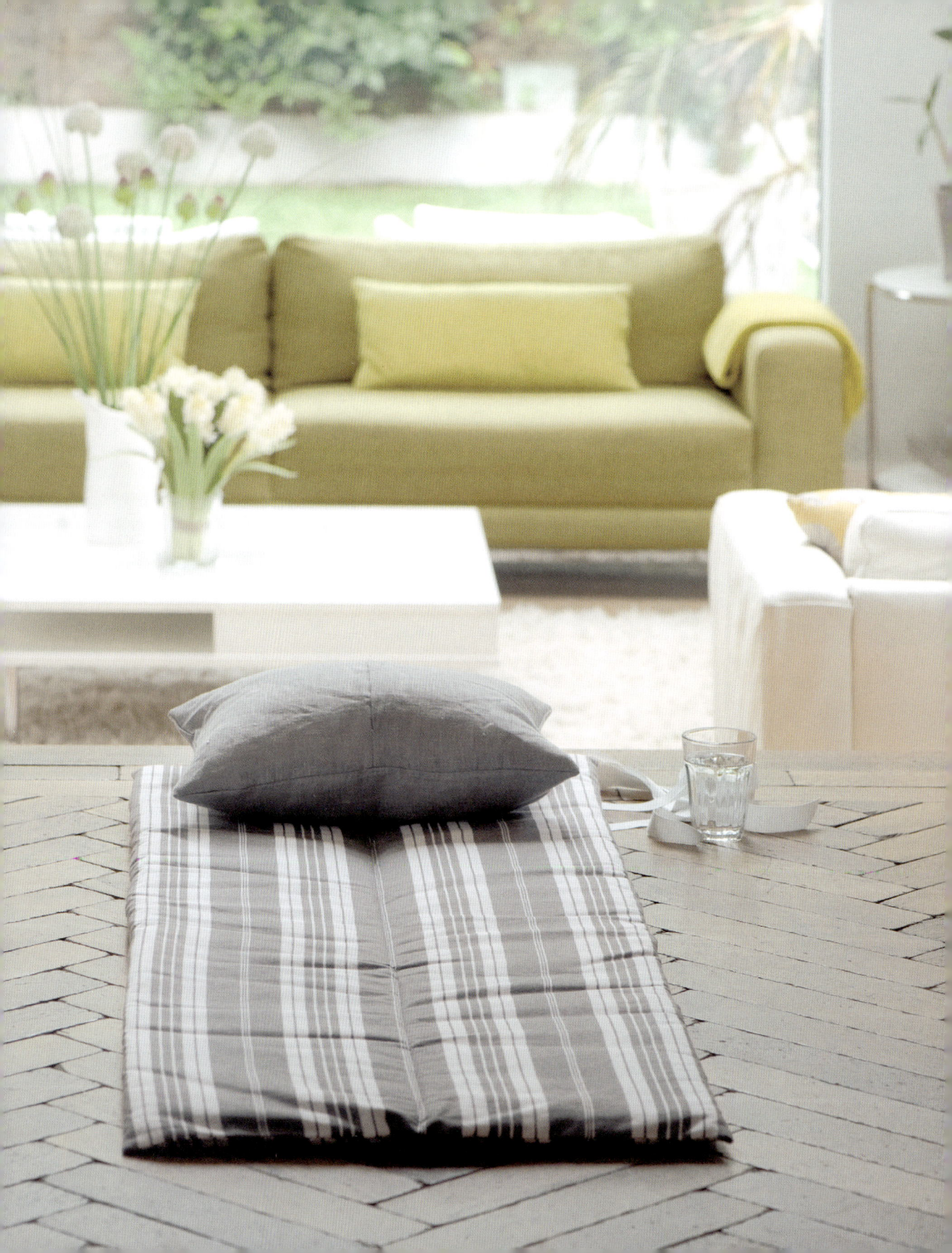

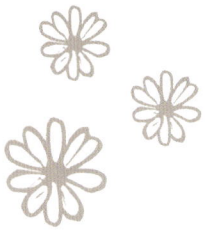

# THE *Wellbeing* Bible

## NOURISH YOUR BODY, MIND, AND SOUL FOR A HEALTHIER, HAPPIER, AND MORE BALANCED LIFE

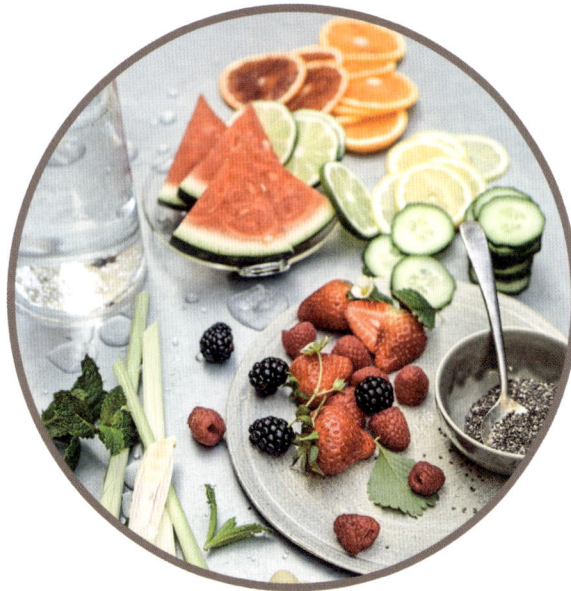

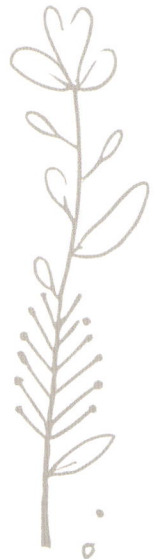

CICO BOOKS

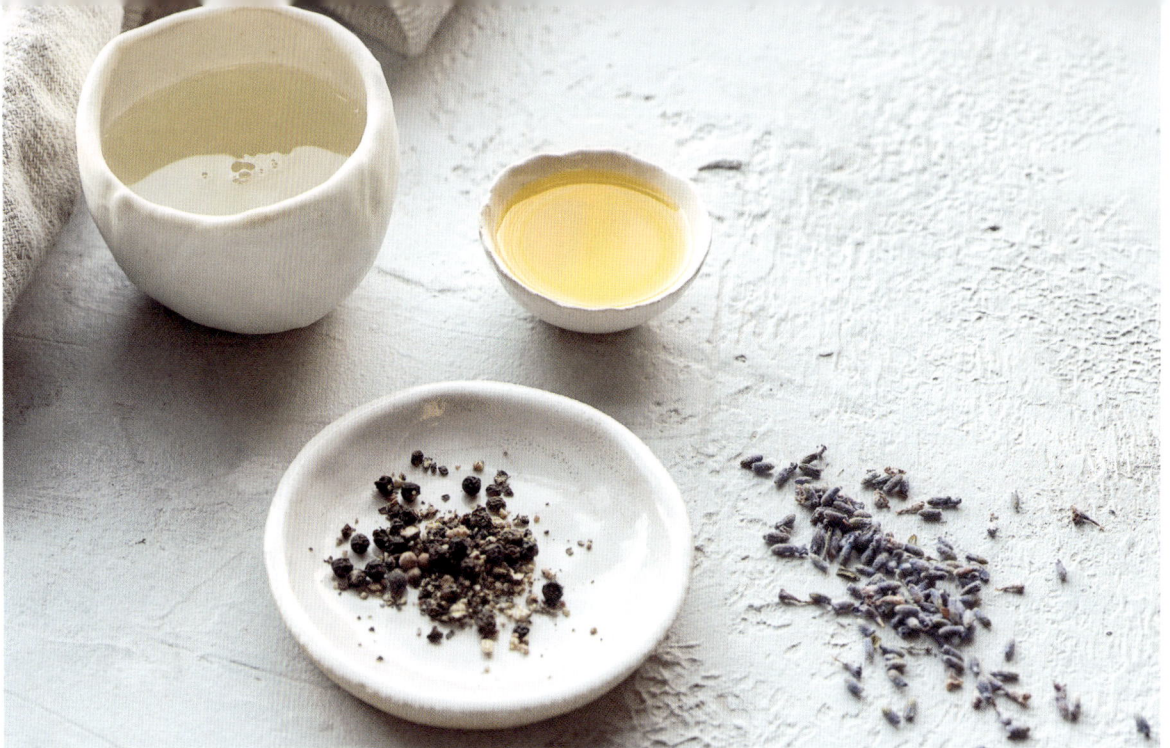

Published in 2026 by CICO Books
An imprint of Ryland Peters & Small Ltd
20–21 Jockey's Fields      1452 Davis Bugg Road
London WC1R 4BW      Warrenton, NC 27589
www.rylandpeters.com
Email: euregulations@rylandpeters.com

Text originally from *Nourish Your Brain Cookbook, Living in the Moment, The Self-healing Revolution, A Year of Living Happily, The Green Cure, Mindfulness and Sleep, The CBD Beauty Book, The Art of Kindness, The Secrets of Happiness,* and *The Power of Gratitude.*

10 9 8 7 6 5 4 3 2 1

A CIP record for this book is available from the British Library. US Library of Congress CIP data has been applied for.

ISBN: 978-1-80065-576-8

Printed in China

Assistant editor: Danielle Rawlings
Senior designer: Emily Breen
Art director: Sally Powell
Creative director: Leslie Harrington
Production manager: Gordana Simakovic
Publishing manager: Carmel Edmonds

The authorized representative in the EEA is Authorised Rep Compliance Ltd., Ground Floor, 71 Lower Baggot Street, Dublin, D01 P593, Ireland
www.arccompliance.com

**Safety note:** If you have food sensitivities or allergies, or are taking any medications, discuss your dietary choices with a health professional or doctor. If you are having a sustained period of difficulty sleeping, consult a health professional or doctor for advice. Please note that while the use of essential oils, CBD oil, and particular practices refer to healing benefits, they are not intended to replace diagnosis of illness or ailments, or healing or medicine. Always consult a health professional or doctor in the case of illness, pregnancy, and other personal sensitivities and conditions. Neither the authors nor the publisher can be held responsible for any claim arising out of the general information, recipes, and practices provided in the book.

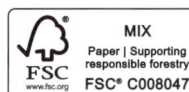

MIX
Paper | Supporting responsible forestry
FSC® C008047
www.fsc.org

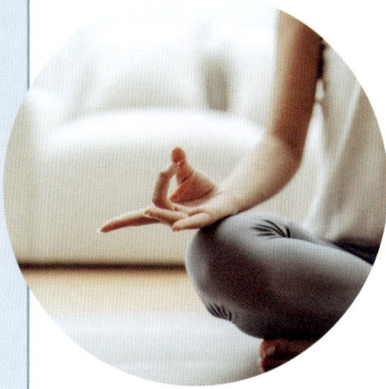
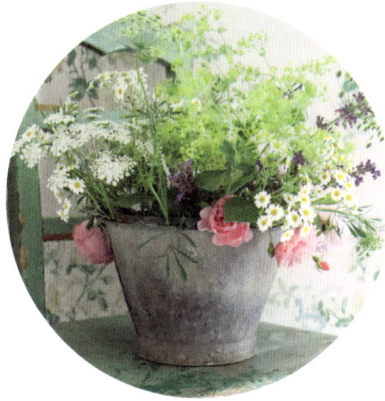
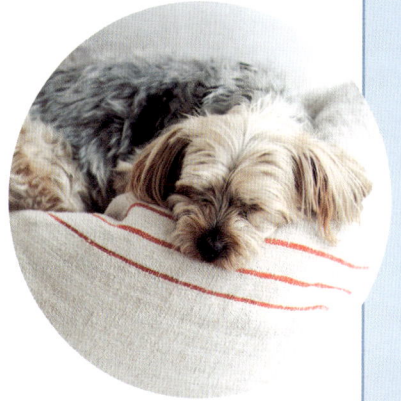

# Contents

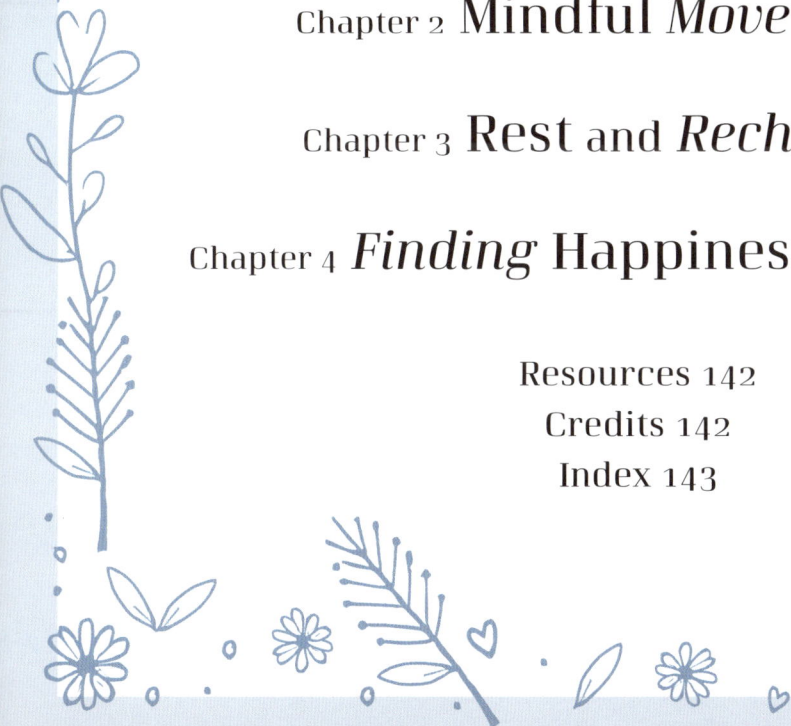

# Introduction

Begin a journey of holistic renewal built on four foundational pillars: how we eat, how we move, how we rest, and how we think and feel.

As you explore each chapter, you'll learn to listen deeply to your body's rhythms and clarity, and cultivate practices rooted in nourishment, presence, and grounded joy. There are no rigid rules—just simple, mindful habits to weave into daily life.

In the first chapter, **Mindful Eating**, we examine how *what* we eat—and *how* we eat—profoundly shapes our wellbeing. It isn't about dieting; it's about bringing gentle awareness to our hunger, enjoyment, and nourishment. Some foods cultivate a thriving microbiome, while others can provoke inflammation. Similarly, our choices influence our energy, mood, and mental clarity. Learn how to recognize foods that uplift you, avoid those that hinder you, and prep meals to harness their full potential.

**Mindful Movement** explores how activities don't have to be strenuous to be transformative. Gentle exercises like yoga, stretching, or walking activate powerful physiological and psychological benefits. Yoga in particular strengthens the body while also calming the mind. Even short, daily sessions—as little as 10–15 minutes, done two or three times weekly—can redirect energy flow, enhance posture, and foster a sense of physical and mental harmony. Through rhythm and breath, you'll unearth a way to feel more alive, centered, and attuned to your body's wisdom.

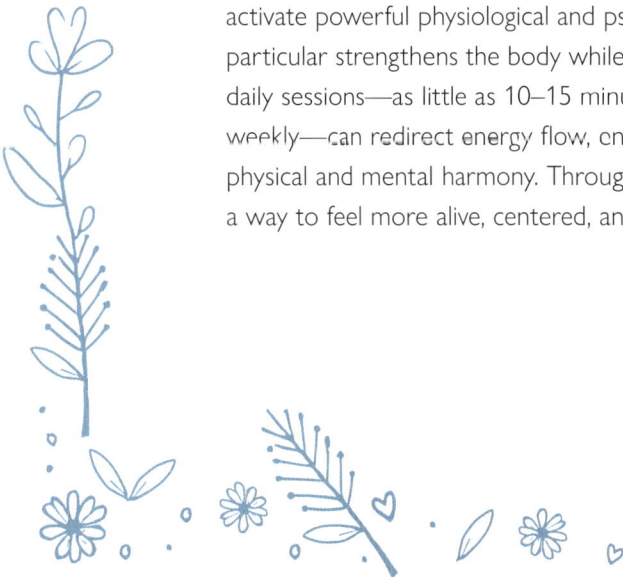

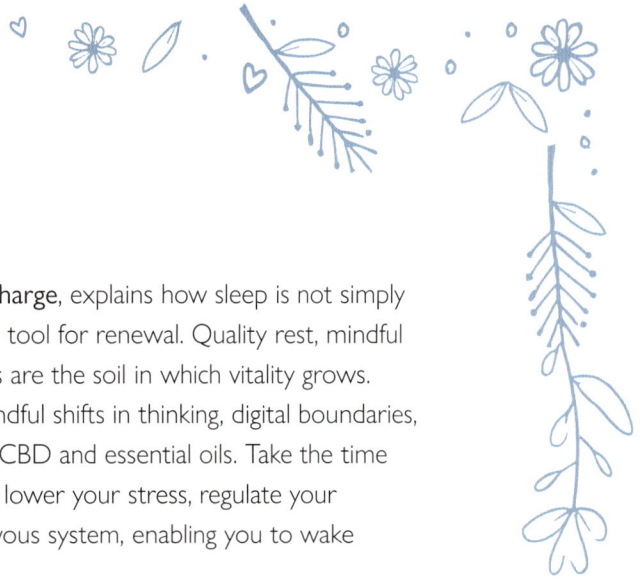

The third chapter, **Rest and Recharge**, explains how sleep is not simply a chore or idleness—it's a powerful tool for renewal. Quality rest, mindful downtime, and restorative practices are the soil in which vitality grows. Nurture that deep rest through mindful shifts in thinking, digital boundaries, calming rituals, and natural aids like CBD and essential oils. Take the time to adjust your routine, and you can lower your stress, regulate your hormones, and rebalance your nervous system, enabling you to wake up restored and resilient.

Finally, lasting happiness doesn't come from chasing extraordinary moments—it grows from small, mindful habits and mental shifts. In **Finding Happiness and Joy**, discover how savoring simple pleasures, kindness toward yourself and others, empathy, embracing your unique self, and daring to try new things can build emotional resilience and reduce stress. As you cultivate calm, practice giving, choose courage over complacency, and dissolve old patterns of negative thinking, joy becomes less about attainment and more about awakening to everyday wonder and connection.

Together, these four foundational pillars offer a practical and inspiring path toward holistic wellbeing, not as a series of one-time fixes, but as everyday habits rooted in presence and nurturing. Each practice reinforces the others: eating well fosters better sleep, which makes movement easier, which in turn uplifts your mood. When you truly listen to your body, you lay the groundwork for a life that feels balanced, connected, and alive. And when your thoughts align with gratitude, curiosity, generosity, and kindness, you open the door to sustained joy and deeper connection with yourself and others.

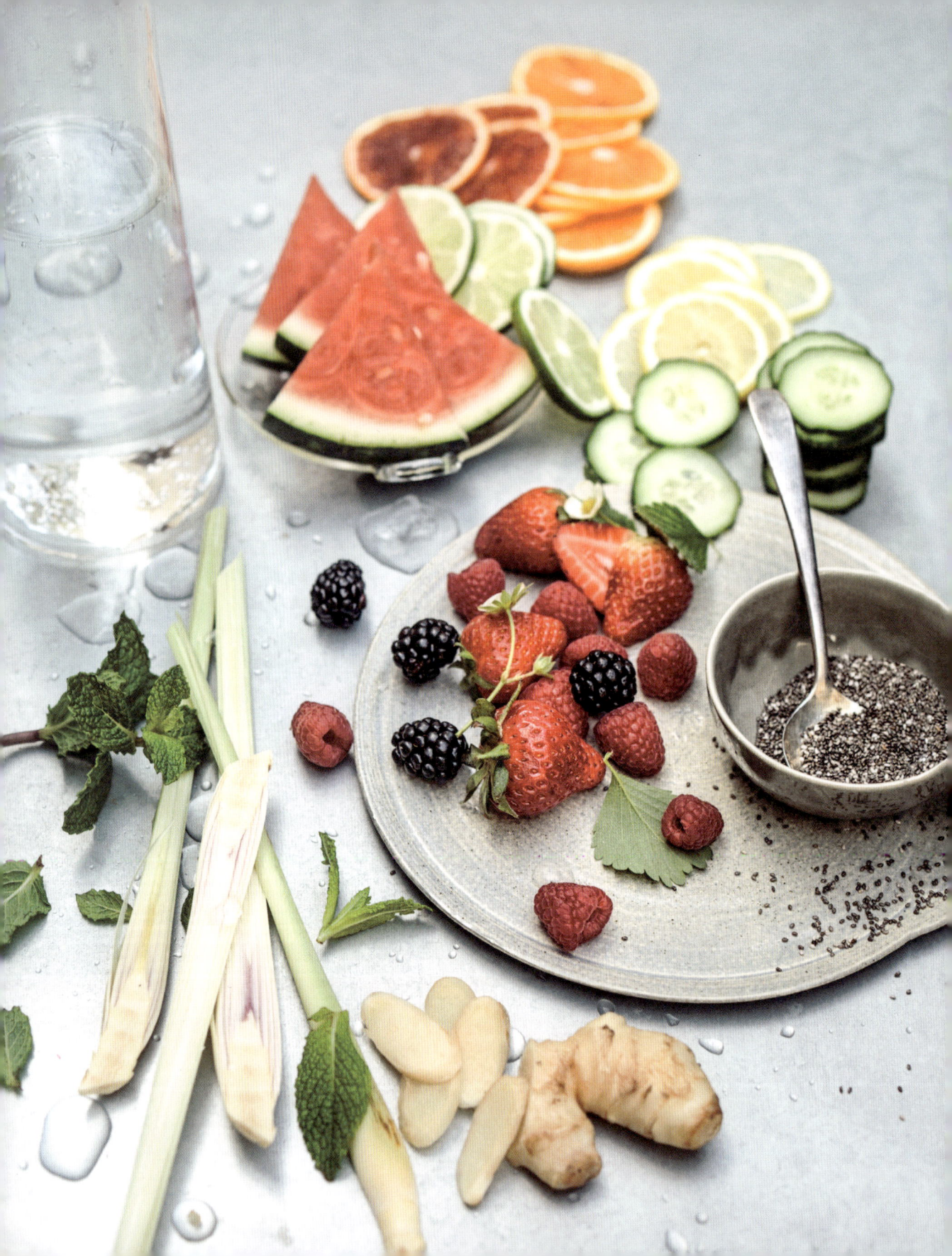

# Chapter 1

# Mindful
# Eating

Transform your relationship with food with
simple changes that will help you achieve
a healthier diet and feel more nourished
in body and mind.

# Our gut–brain connection

Our brain and gut are closely interconnected in terms of our senses, biological functions, emotions, and moods.

You know what it feels like when you smell freshly baked cookies and your mouth waters. You also know what it is like when you have a gut feeling about a situation, or when you feel sick to your stomach when you are very upset. You also know how emotionally satisfied you can feel after you have enjoyed a delicious meal with loved ones.

Every piece of food we consume and every stressful thought we have affects our brain directly, in both gut and head. Both "brains" need to be nourished if we wish to perform well, maintain mental energy, and stay emotionally balanced.

Unhealthy processed or junk foods irritate the stomach—and they will irritate the brain, too. They contribute to inflammation in the gut and brain, and over time that can contribute to many illnesses, including autoimmune diseases (see page 20), developmental problems in children, painful joints, cognitive difficulties, and degenerative neurological diseases in adults.

## The science behind it

Time for a little anatomy: Our two "brains" are closely connected by a complex nervous system that relies heavily on the vagus nerve. This large nerve is like the captain of the ship, conducting information back and forth from the brain to all the organs and glands that are involved with our digestion, breathing, and heart function. It is also known as the gut–brain axis.

The digestive tract is like a rubber tube that runs from the mouth down to the anus. Millions of nerves are embedded in its walls, and that is why we can feel pain and other symptoms if we have trouble digesting certain foods. This network of nerves is the enteric nervous system, and it is also known as the "second brain." The gut tube has a mucosal lining of gut-associated lymphoid tissue that forms a large part of our immune system. Its role is to provide a protective boundary between the outside world and our inside body. It is often said that all disease begins in the gut.

When foods move from the mouth through the digestive tract, many different hormones, nerves, and digestive enzymes are called to action by the gut–brain in our innards. Digestion requires a lot of energy; after all, it is the biggest driver of our metabolic fire. Too much stress in daily life, and a lack of nutrients such as zinc, affects the body's ability to release stomach acid and enzymes that are essential for healthy digestion and the absorption of nutrients. Both too much and too little stomach acid is a problem.

Any undigested food that putrefies and ferments in the stomach invites harmful microbes and yeasts to feast on it. At the same time, you may be noticing digestive symptoms such as acid reflux, gastric inflammation, bloating, excessive gas, or constipation, while your mind is experiencing ADHD (attention deficit hyperactivity disorder), anxiety, brain fog, and funky moods. You might also experience itchy skin, sleep difficulties, or tightness in the chest (do consult a cardiologist if you have this last symptom, to rule out cardiovascular problems). In addition, any difficulties with elimination or excessive bowel activity are an indicator of digestive troubles that can originate higher up.

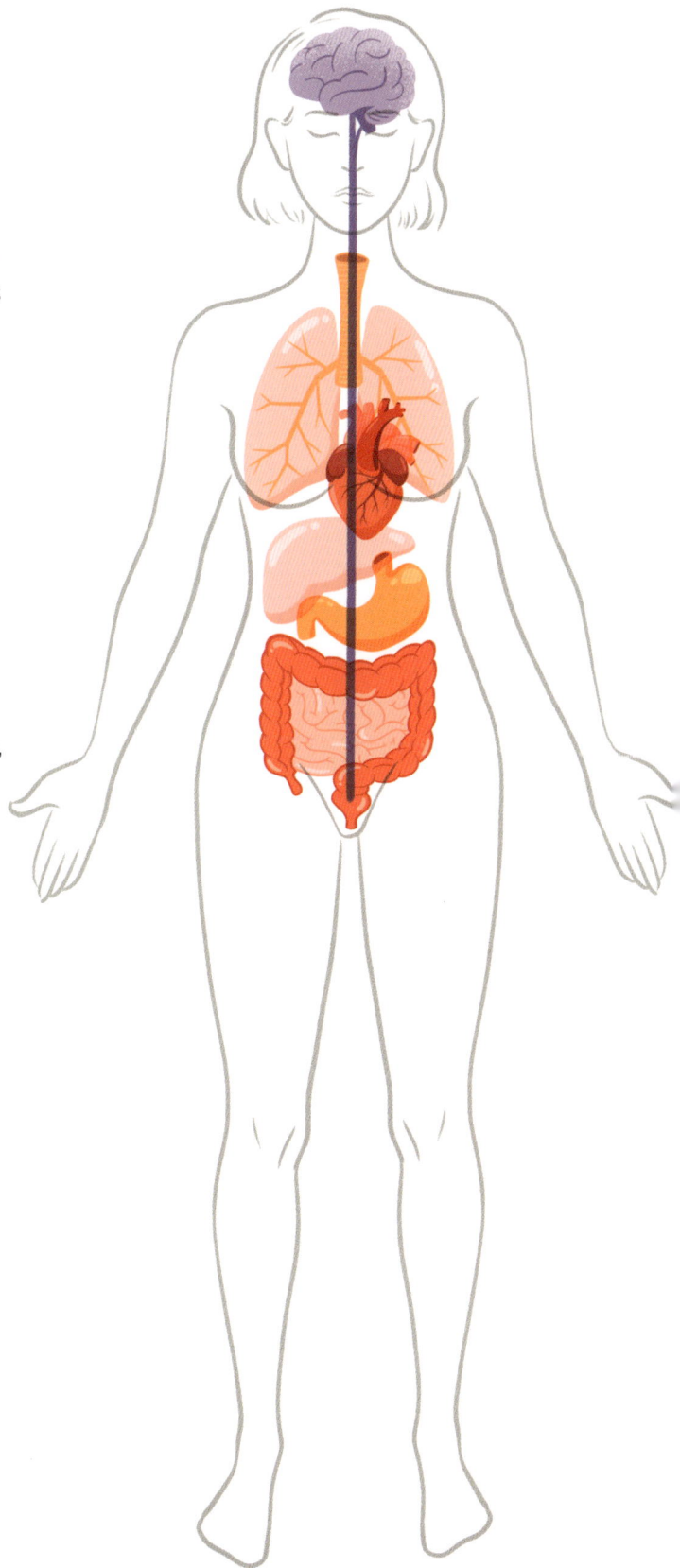

Right: The vagus nerve conducts information back and forth from the brain to the rest of the body. This is a simplified diagram—in reality, the nerve descends from the brain as a pair of nerves and branches out throughout the body.

# The basics for a healthy brain

While we go about our busy lives juggling home and work commitments throughout the day, we hardly think about the most important organ in our head—our brain.

Different areas of our brain allow us to hear sounds, smell aromas, think and speak freely, move our limbs, breathe, memorize experiences, interpret information from the outside world, and learn new things that are useful in our lives. Think about it: If you stub your little toe, it hurts. Your brain knows that, too. If you walk into a surprise birthday party and your heart pumps with excitement, your brain is charged up, too, with excitable brain chemicals and adrenaline. All are simple examples of how the brain is implicated in every situation.

Even at night, our brain does not rest when we do. While we sleep, the brain ensures that we breathe and maintain steady blood sugar, and that our heart keeps beating. It also processes and stores information gathered during the busy day, reinforcing our memory. Not only that, but "housecleaning" in the brain also occurs at night. While we sleep, the brain shrinks slightly, and the lymphatic fluid can sweep out accumulated toxins that contribute to inflammation and premature aging.

## Food for thought

How we manage stress, beginning with a healthy eating, exercise, and sleep strategy, will have a great impact on the long-term wellness of our brain. Consider, for example, that a deficiency of vitamin B12 is associated with dementia and tingling sensations in feet and fingers. Every day, every meal, it matters what and when we eat, as our blood-sugar balance and brain energy depend on it. A nutrient-deprived brain ages faster.

It is particularly important to nourish a developing brain in a young child, and an aging brain in the later stages of life, when often more nutrients are needed than are supplied in the daily diet. Sadly, foods today contain much lower levels of vitamins and minerals than the foods our grandparents ate. Skipping meals creates an energy crisis, depriving the brain of the energy it needs if we are to think clearly.

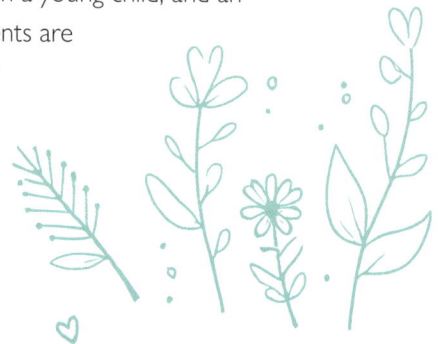

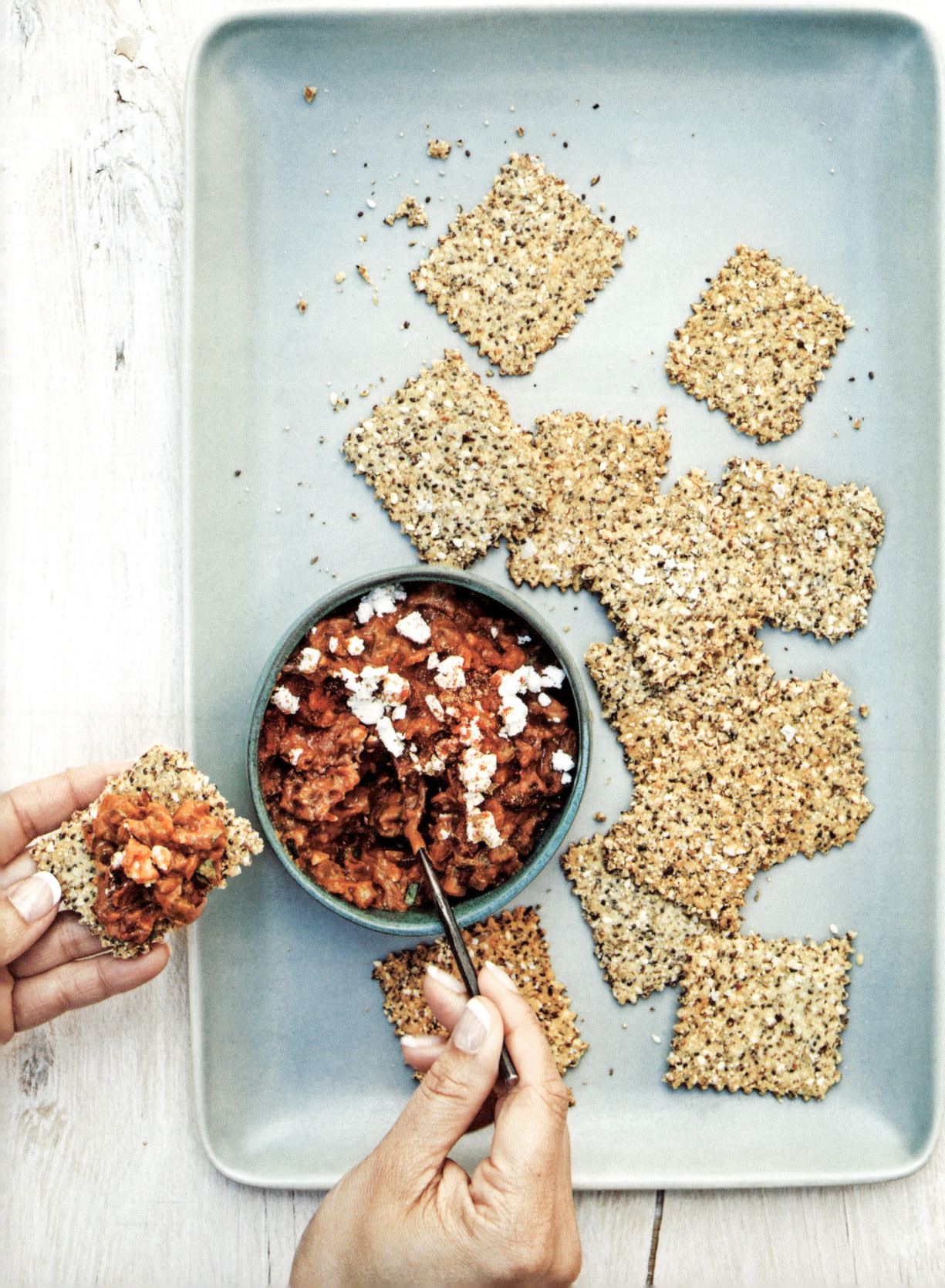

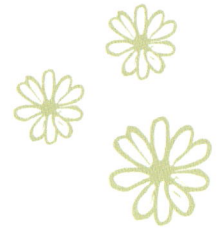

# Gut flora, probiotics, and prebiotics

A diverse gut flora plays an important part in our resilience (physical, mental, and emotional), our outlook on life, and our ability to maintain a rational mindset.

Think of your gut flora as an internal soil and garden that you carry around with you wherever you go. This ecology becomes a lifelong template that promotes or decreases our physical health and mental wellbeing. It needs tending, just like the vegetable patch in a backyard. What we eat affects our microbes and our moods directly.

Prebiotics are like a fertilizer for the good microbes in our gut—they optimize the balance of our bowel flora and absorption of nutrients. They consist of the insoluble fiber in fruits, vegetables, and grains and are fermented and converted into short-chain fatty acids called butyrate. Butyrate is often deficient in many chronic illnesses and autoimmune diseases, including colitis and irritable bowel syndrome (IBS), so it's important to have it.

Probiotics are live bacteria that are part of the body's microbiome, and they feed on prebiotics. So the more fiber-rich foods we incorporate into our diet, the happier our probiotics are. Well-known examples of probiotics are species of *Lactobacillus*, including *L. bifidus* and *L. acidophilus*, and a healthy yeast called *Saccharomyces boulardii*.

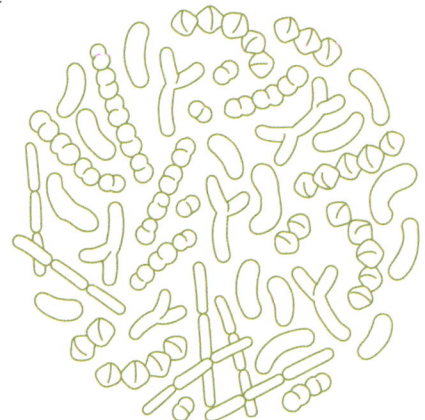

Right: The microbes in our gut (known as the microbiata) are like busy construction workers on a work site.

## FOOD FOR A FLOURISHING GUT FLORA

Examples of prebiotics in food include the inulin in bananas and fiber in garlic, leeks, onions, avocados, legumes, coconut flakes, and guar gum (found in many processed foods). Additional prebiotic supplementation includes fructooligosaccharides (FOS), psyllium husk, and acacia.

Probiotics occur naturally in cultured and fermented foods such as kefir, yogurt, sauerkraut, tempeh, miso, and pickles. It is also possible to supplement your diet with soil- and spore-based probiotics. These beneficial microbes add to the diversity within an individual's gut flora, but you should consult with a health practitioner to discuss which probiotic choice is best for you.

Dark leafy greens, multicolored vegetables, fermented foods, and healthy fats from nuts, seeds, pasture-raised animals, and fish, also help our body to get rid of the toxins that we are exposed to daily.

Fermented foods and drinks such as sauerkraut, kimchee, kombucha, and kefir encourage health-supporting bacteria and yeasts in our gut, but are not in the mainstream diet. We need them, however, since they play an important part in maintaining our mood and energy.

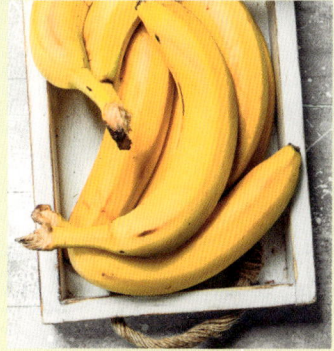

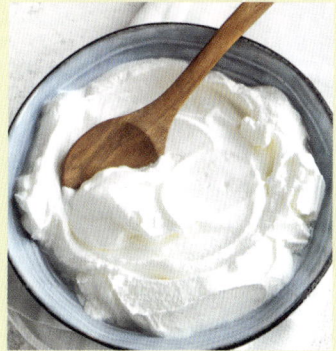

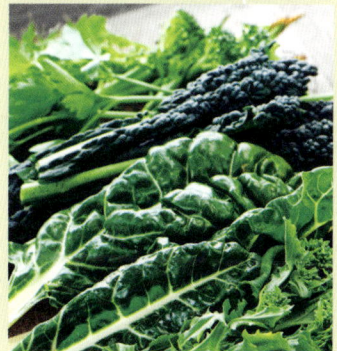

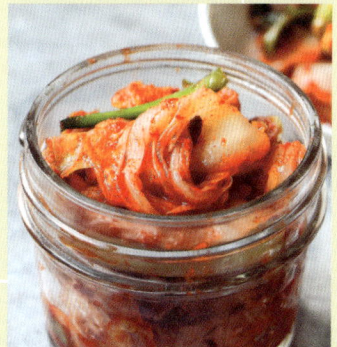

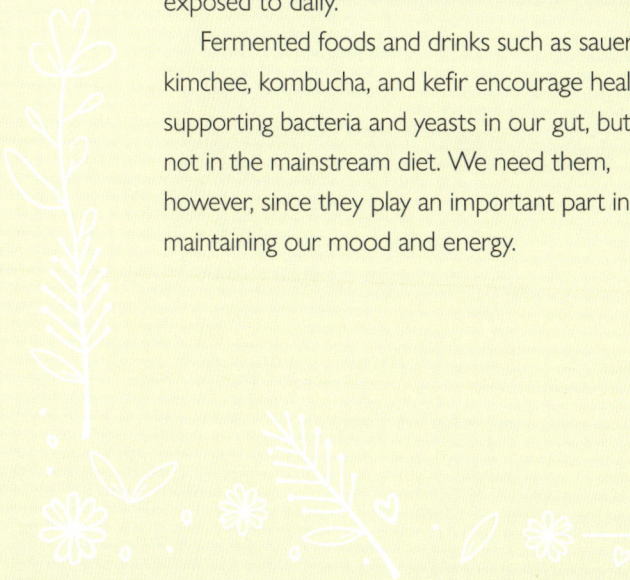

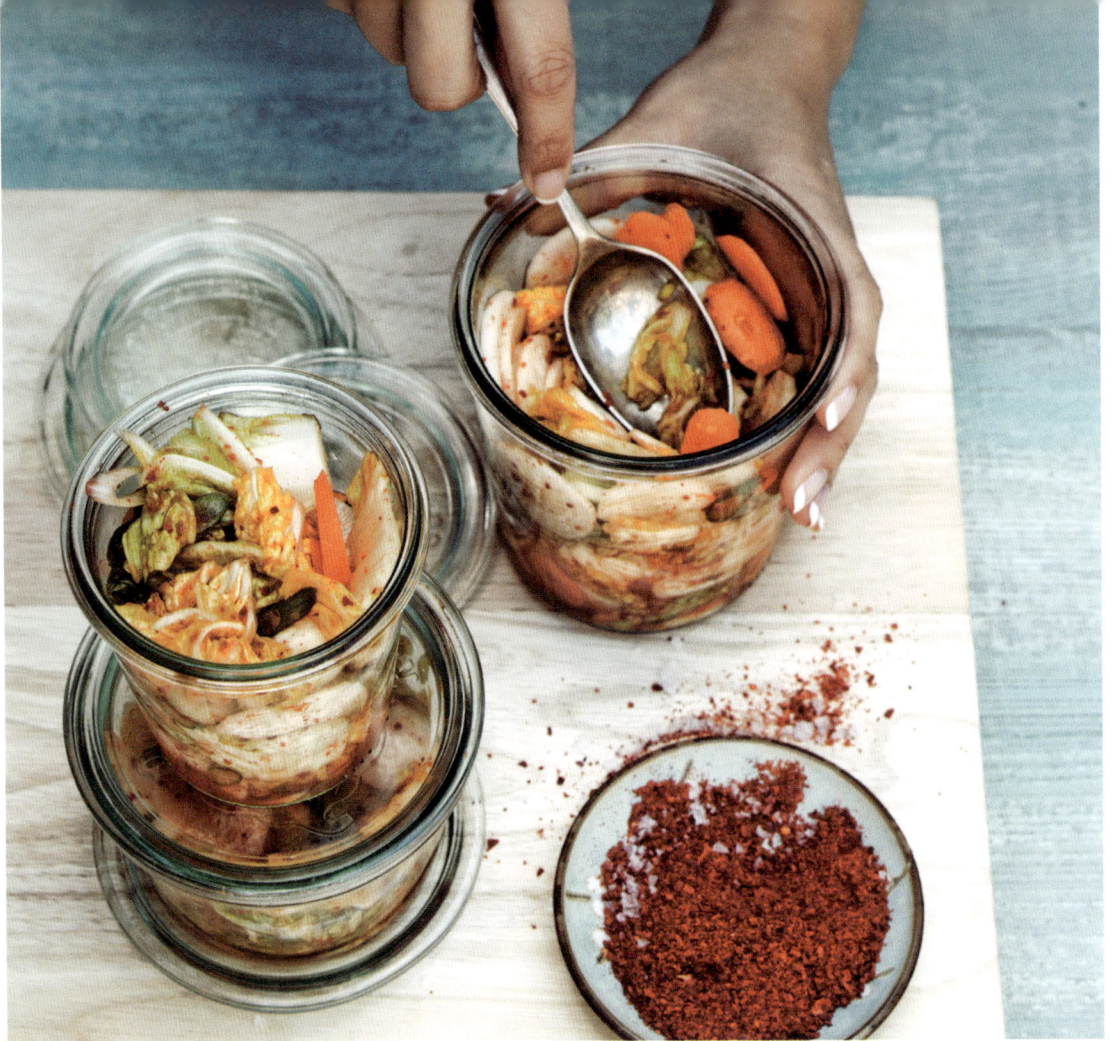

# How to nourish
# your gut and brain

Improper eating can result in your memory and cognitive function diminishing, meaning it's so important to pay attention to what you eat. Here is a list of essentials that make a great foundation for your brain-health pantry.

## Fermented foods

These make the nutrients in food easier to absorb and provide a variety of health-supporting probiotics. Try kefir in a smoothie, sauerkraut with grilled chicken, or pickles as a twist to your salad.

## Fruity fruit and varied veggies

The enzymes, minerals, and vitamins found in raw foods, salads, and smoothies help to heal tissues, and are part of various biochemical processes that affect our energy and our ability to handle the stress of daily life. Vitamins A, K, and C in these foods help to heal a leaky gut (see page 20). The more colors on your plate, the better you can provide your brain and body a variety of phytonutrients:

- Tannins are the water-soluble phenols found in grape skins, cocoa, tea, sage, cranberries, and red wine. They have astringent properties, and their health benefits include the inhibition of plaque formation on teeth, the healing of wounds, and the alleviation of gastritis and diarrhea.
- Flavonoids are phytonutrients that have anti-cancer, heart healthy, and brain-healthy properties, while also improving memory and microcirculation in the brain. They are found in plant-based foods and determine the color of the vegetable or fruit: the darker the color, the better, as in blueberries, purple grapes, blackberries, parsley, black beans, capers, and green tea.
- Organosulfur compounds are essential minerals needed for the detoxification pathways that play an important role in our ability to eliminate environmental toxins, chemical estrogens in plastics, and infections. A lack of these may increase our risk of cancer of the reproductive organs. Sulfur-containing foods include eggs (especially the white), meat, and vegetables such as broccoli, cabbage, bok choy (pak choi), turnips, onions, garlic, and leeks.
- Resveratrol is a potent antioxidant and anti-inflammatory found in certain fruits, red wine, and cocoa. It increases microcirculation in the brain and heart, and is a memory, vision, and immune modulator. Resveratrol can cross the blood–brain barrier. (Incidentally, Japanese knotweed, a great source of resveratrol, is used in botanical treatments for Lyme disease.)

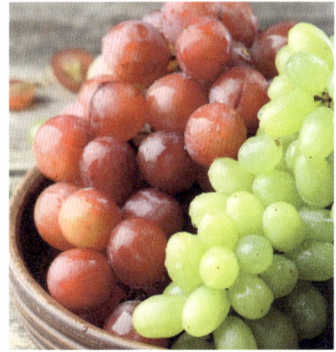

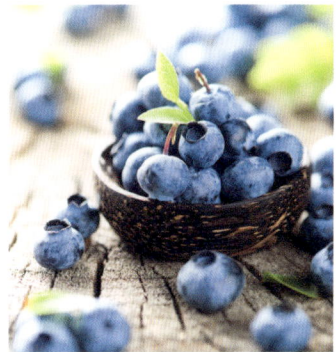

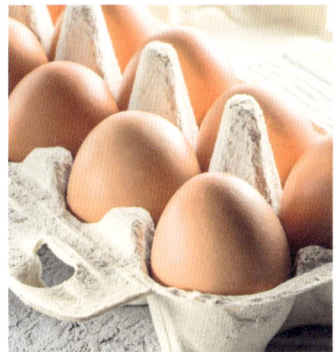

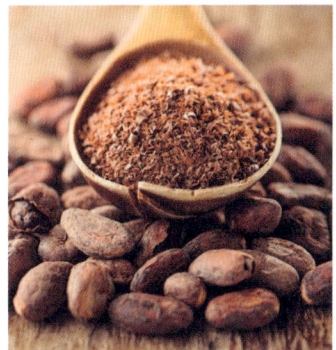

## Eat whole

The skin of organic fruit also has health benefits, but this is not widely known. Grate some fresh orange peel over your salad or breakfast bowl for detox agents in the quercetin and limonene family. If you are going to eat fruit skins it is doubly important that you go organic, since most pesticides are contained within the skin—and do wash it well.

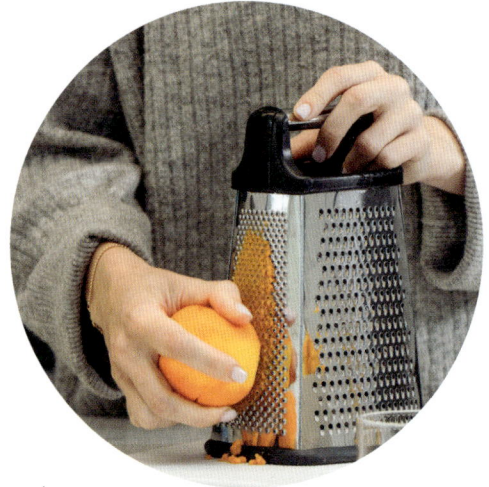

## Healing herbs

We infuse herbal medicine into our home-cooked meals when we add rosemary, thyme, oregano, sage, bay leaf, savory, marjoram, basil, parsley, or cilantro (coriander). Herbs will lift the taste of any hot dish, or chop some fresh herbs as a decorative anti-inflammatory addition to your summer salad.

## Spice it up

Cumin, cloves, cayenne pepper, paprika, cinnamon, and more are staples in a spice rack for a healthy kitchen. Spices have great nutritional and medicinal value and improve our cognition and memory. Curcumin, the active component of golden turmeric, has been shown to encourage the growth of new neurons while also altering degenerative processes in the brain. That is exciting news! Curcumin has powerful anti-aging, anti-inflammatory, and anti-cancer properties, and has been used in traditional medicine for many centuries. Today many use a daily turmeric supplement against pain and inflammation, although not everyone tolerates turmeric. (Before using any supplementation do check with your doctor if you are on blood-thinning medication, or have gallbladder trouble or diabetes.)

## Enjoy a cup of tea

Choose any herbal tea or elixir and add a sprig of lemongrass or rosemary to connect with your sense of wellness. It has been established that green tea contains the phytonutrient EGCG (epigallocatechin-3-gallate), which helps the body to get rid of toxins, has anti-cancer properties, and is anti-inflammatory. All that in one cup of tea!

## Daily detox

Garlic, which contains the active phytonutrient allicin, has the potential to lower blood pressure while providing sulfur for detox. Foods such as broccoli, cabbages, radishes, and dark leafy greens are also dense in phytonutrients. They contain a compound called sulforaphane, which promotes the elimination of harmful chemicals, chemical estrogens in plastics, and environmental toxins. The more toxins we can get rid of, the more we will protect our brain in the long term.

## Fabulous fiber

High-fiber foods such as bananas, yams, leeks, avocado, cassava, artichoke, asparagus, fennel, okra, chickpeas, split peas, and couscous are all food sources for microbes. They get their energy by fermenting the fiber in these whole foods. It's important to feed our friendly microbes, so that they can feed our brain.

## Beneficial broth (stock)

The elixir for "leaky gut syndrome" (see page 20) can be found in chicken (especially the gelatin-rich chicken feet and also pigs' feet), beef, lamb, fish, and their bones. The amino acids, trace minerals, gelatin, and collagen they contain improve digestion, help to heal mucosal linings in the brain and gut, and provide overall nourishment.

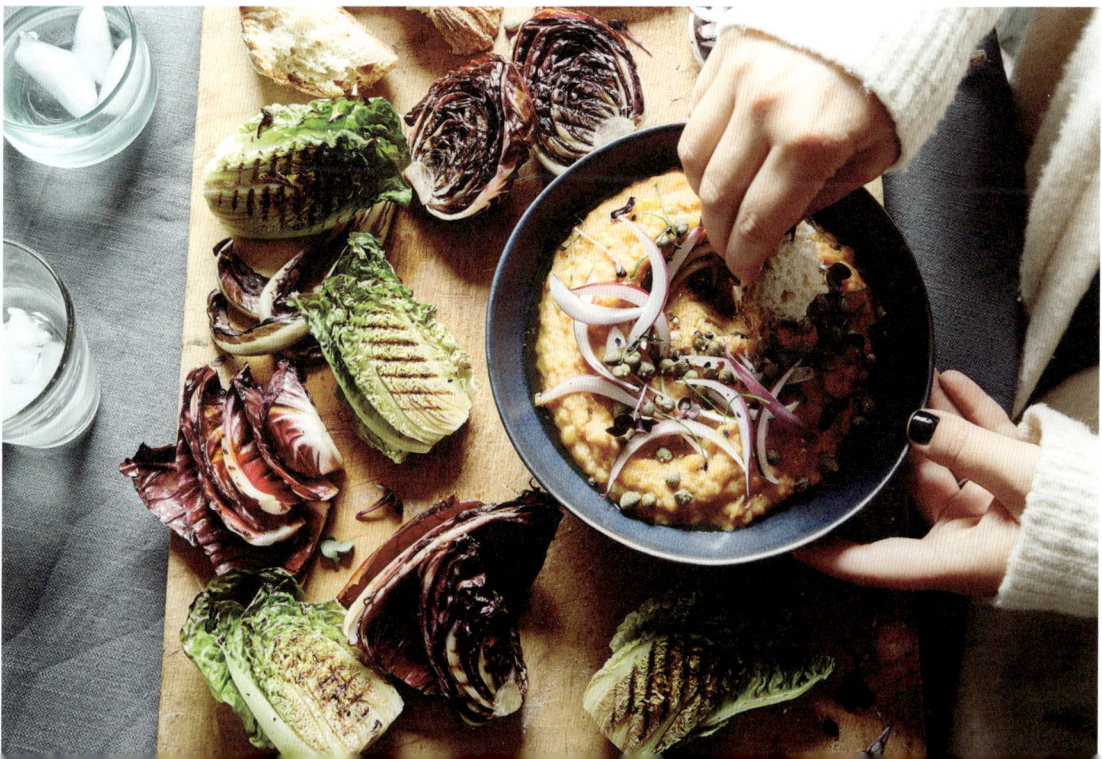

# Easing inflammation

If the mucosal barrier in the gut is breached or becomes porous in places, intestinal semi-permeability arises, commonly known as "leaky gut." This breach triggers an inflammatory process that can have far-reaching effects if the body is not able to heal it within a few days.

Pesticides, especially glyphosate, in commercial foods cause or contribute to a leaky gut, which is associated with sustained inflammation. All can leave you constantly fatigued and weakened with multiple food sensitivities and trouble with learning, memory, and cognitive function. If a leaky gut continues unchecked for months or even years, food particles, allergens, toxins, and infectious agents can gain entry into the body. This wreaks havoc, as the immune system becomes hyper-vigilant and cannot distinguish self from non-self. This is the basis of most autoimmune diseases. Healthy tissues in the body will be attacked, and this can affect the brain, thyroid, pancreas, colon, joints, skin, and more. We can experience headaches, pain, insomnia, and anxiety as our stress meter is dialed up.

Chronic inflammation associated with a leaky gut and leaky brain also plays a role in many neurological diseases, chronic pain, migraines, and psychiatric conditions. Consider it as an ongoing low-grade irritant to the body that diminishes our resilience and makes us age faster on the outside and the inside. Even though we might not be aware of it, the immune system is irritated by the accumulation of environmental toxins, lack of sleep, medications, emotional, financial, or work stress, personal relationship troubles, and more. All contribute to low-grade sustained inflammation that adversely affects blood-sugar balance, energy production, cognition, mood, and memory, and it depletes our nutrient reserves, thyroid function, and reproductive hormones.

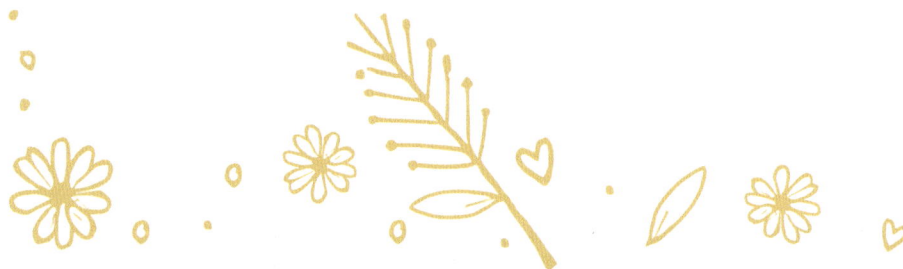

## TOP 15 FOODS FOR LOWERING INFLAMMATION

To remedy inflammation, avoid processed ingredients, such as trans fats, food coloring, chemicals, and flavorings. Instead, stock up on the following:

- Papaya
- Blueberries
- Ginger
- Avocado
- Rosemary
- Bone broth (stock)
- Turmeric
- Celery
- Dark leafy greens
- Beets (beetroot) and tops
- Fatty wild-caught fish
- Garlic
- Chamomile
- Cod-liver oil
- Okra

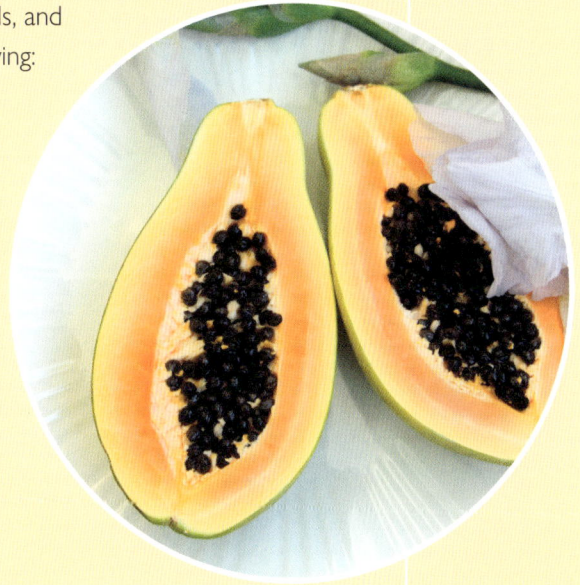

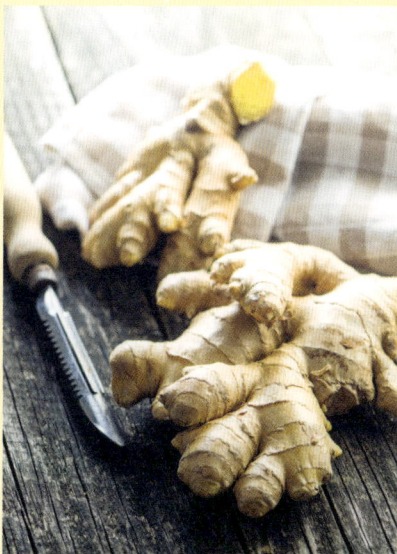

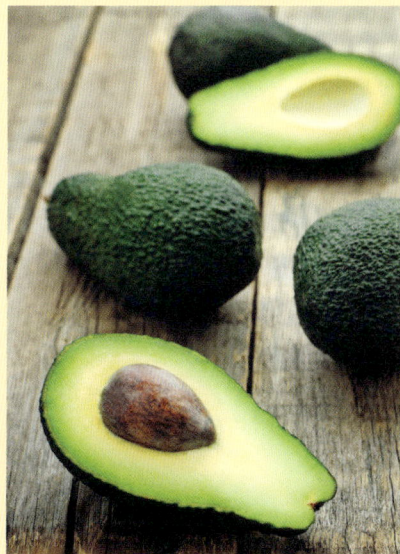

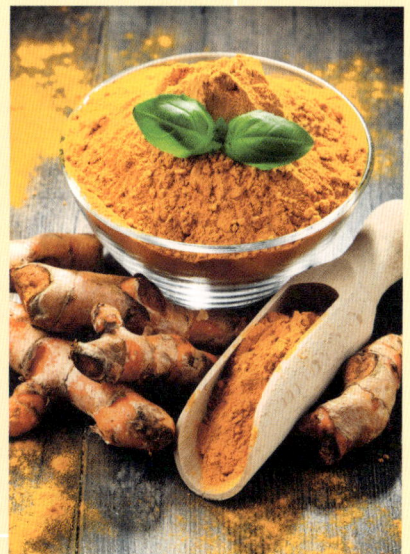

# Choosing gut-friendly foods

Sometimes it's difficult to know which foods are best for you and which to avoid. This information will help you seek out those which are friendly toward your gut—and those that are not so friendly.

## Good foods that combat disease

- Multicolored organic vegetables and fruit provide an array of vitamins and minerals needed for the healthy function of the brain. These include carrots, broccoli, celery, avocado, salads, dark leafy greens, beets (beetroot), onions, garlic, blueberries, pineapple, and grapes.
- Free-range poultry, pasture-raised animals, organ meats, and byproducts (such as eggs, butter, chicken fat). It's helpful to include homemade broth (stock) and gelatin as bioavailable protein sources for brain and mood health.
- Nuts and seeds, ideally soaked, drained, and dried. These provide a wide array of omega-3 and unrefined omega-6 oils that support healthy brain membranes and lower overall inflammation. Brazil nuts, walnuts, almonds, pecans, pistachios, macadamias, and hazelnuts are fine choices.

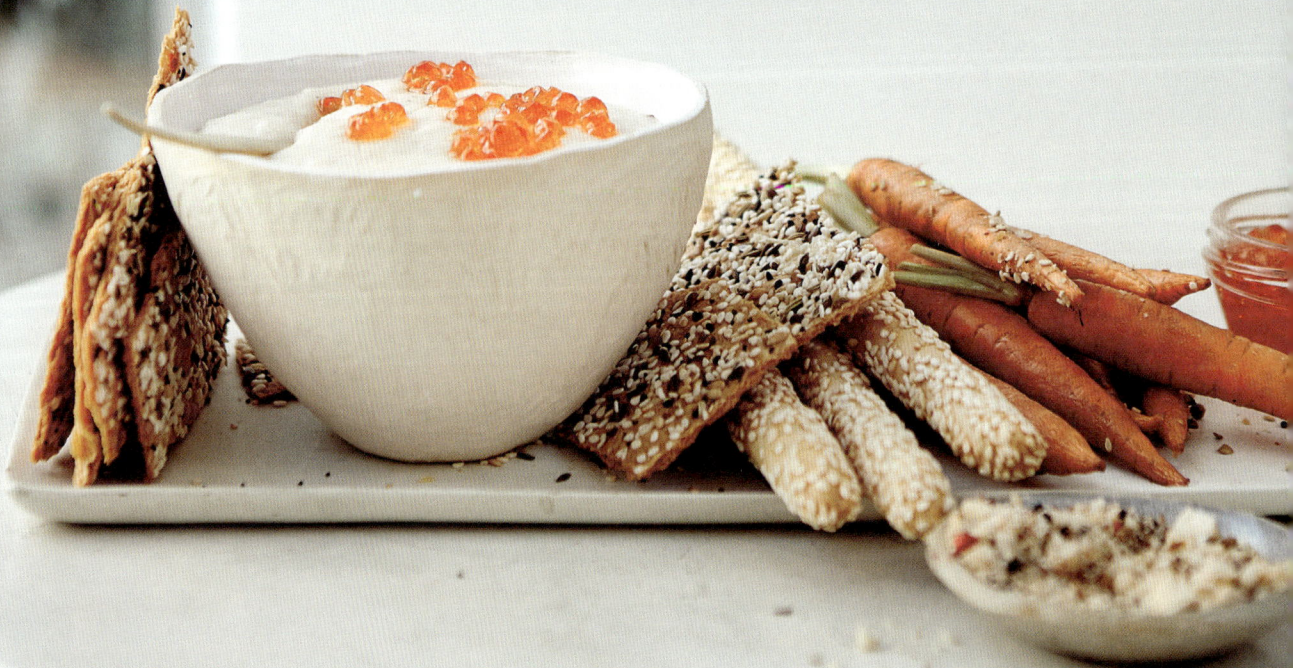

- "Healthy brain" fats and oils, including cold-pressed olive oil, organic butter, ghee, coconut oil, lard, evening primrose oil, palm oil (from sustainable sources), and unrefined safflower, sunflower, walnut, and avocado oils. Naturally occurring sugars in fruit, raw honey and maple syrup (preferably local), and molasses (stevia is acceptable).
- Home-cooked oatmeal (porridge) or grains, preferably stoneground, rich in fiber and B vitamins. Steel-cut oats or barley are favorites, but also investigate buckwheat groats, quinoa, millet, and amaranth. Chia, coconut flakes, and hemp seeds can be mixed with nuts and fruit.
- Purified/filtered/spring water, ideally in glass bottles. Clean, mineral-rich water flushes out toxins from the brain.
- Home-squeezed fruit and vegetable juices contain natural fiber that prevents a spike in blood sugar. Choose just one fruit serving if you juice, such as a cup of mixed berries or one banana, and add a source of protein and fat to complement it.
- Slow-cooking: baked, crockpot, roasted, sautéed, low-heat grilling, steamed food preparation.
- Cold-water fish that lower inflammation. These include anchovies, cod, halibut, wild salmon, herring, and sardines, all of which contain healthy omega-3 fats. (Smaller fish are less contaminated with mercury.)

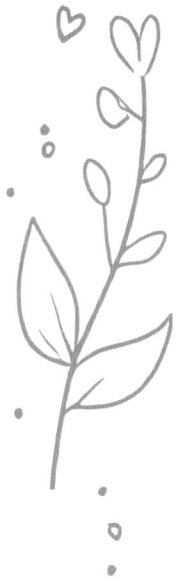

## Foods to avoid

- Commercially processed foods with a long shelf life, excessive refined sugars, and sodium.
- All factory-farmed animal proteins, processed breakfast and luncheon meats, and commercial poultry.
- Rancid processed nuts with excessive sodium, often stored in moldy conditions that contribute to mold toxicity symptoms.
- Excessive fats, and all fast and deep-fried foods.
- Artificial sweeteners of any kind.
- Processed cereals from refined grains (GMO crops in the USA) that are low in fiber with the chemical BHT (butylated hydroxytoluene).
- Sodas, diet drinks, and synthetic flavored water.
- Processed concentrated fruit juices, even if organic.
- Tuna, king mackerel, and swordfish that contain high levels of mercury.

# Improving energy, stable moods, and focus

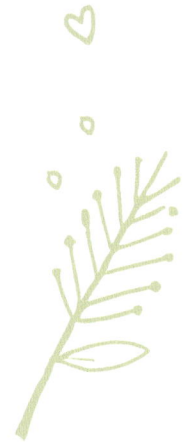

What we eat and when we eat directly affects how well we function—and that is empowering to know. All day long our brain needs a steady stream of energy from food for optimal cognition, memory, attention, happy thoughts, and a stable mood.

## Protein

For a productive and high-performing day, include a good source of protein in your breakfast. A lack of protein in the diet affects our blood-sugar balance, mood, and concentration. If you have a smaller appetite in the morning, you might prefer oatmeal (porridge), a bowl of yogurt, or a smoothie. If you have a large appetite and respond well to a hearty breakfast, enjoy an omelet, or add avocado and protein powder to your smoothie.

A vegetarian or vegan diet can insidiously induce deficiencies in fat-soluble vitamin A, B12, zinc, choline (a macronutrient that is needed for brain and nerve function), cholesterol, and amino acids. This can contribute to depressed moods as well as affecting other functions, such as bone health challenges, muscle wasting, and infertility. It is particularly important for those who follow these diets to create a good mix of protein by combining different protein groups in each meal. It is worth considering supplementation with minerals, vitamin B12, and fat soluble vitamins A, D, and K.

## Sugar

Scientific evidence shows that eating too many sugary foods contributes to an accumulation of harmful molecules, called advanced glycation end products (AGEs). These promote harmful free-radical damage from toxic molecules—think of it as internal rusting. Over many years, they contribute to low-grade brain inflammation that is associated with adult neurodegenerative diseases such as dementia, MS, Parkinson's disease, and Alzheimer's.

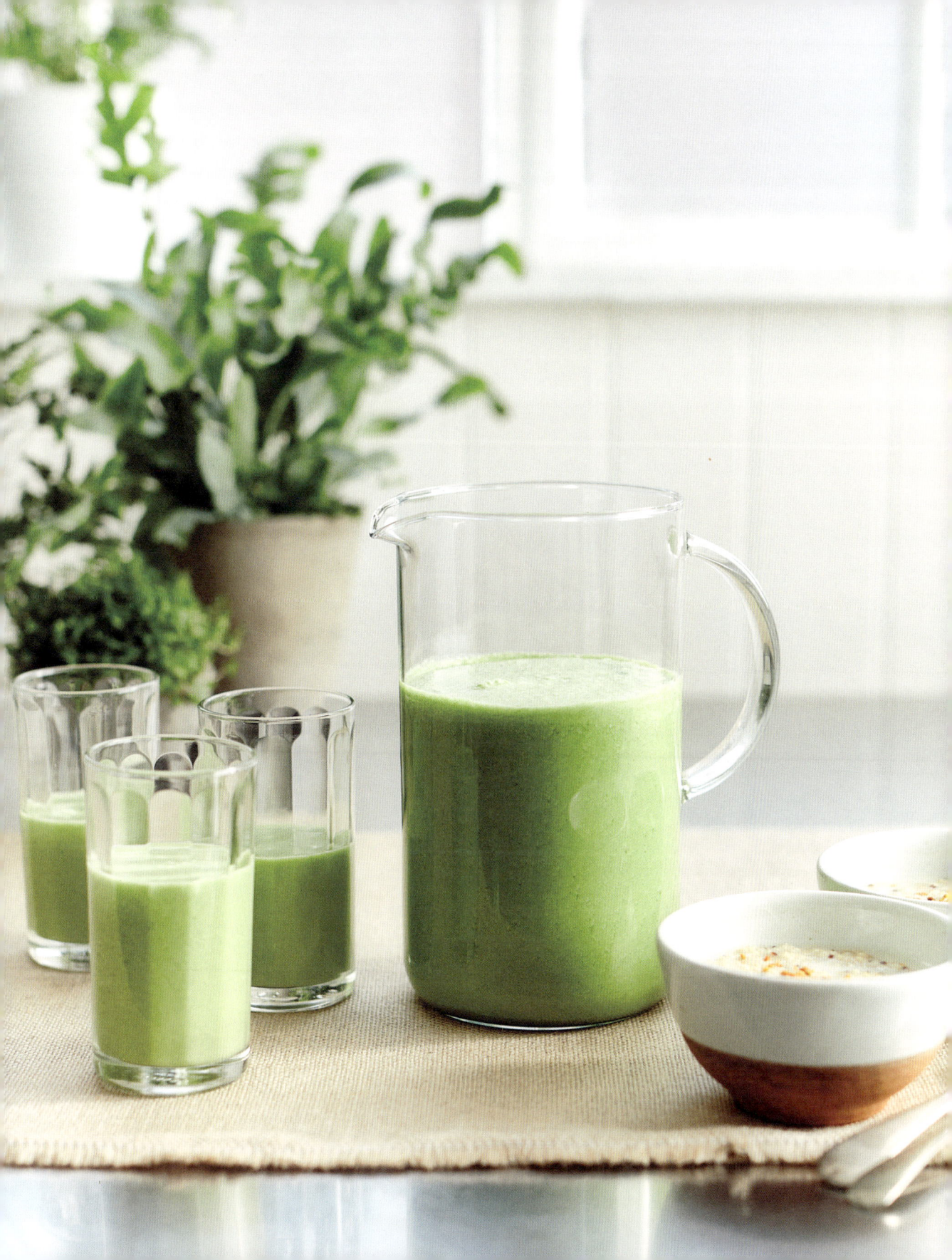

# TOP 20 BENEFICIAL (ORGANIC) FOODS

To get through a busy day, we all need a brain that is sharp and focused, whether as kids going to school, adults at work, or simply in order to play a fun game of chess with a friend. These lovely treats will do just the trick.

- Dark leafy vegetables, such as spinach* and kale
- Purple grapes
- Multicolored berries
- Avocado*
- Coconut oil
- Free-range egg yolks*
- Extra-virgin olive oil
- Wild salmon (smoked, cooked, or canned)*
- Rosemary
- Turmeric
- Gingko tea
- Green tea extract
- Brahmi tea
- Grapeseed oil
- Walnuts*
- Cod-liver oil
- Butter*
- Dark chocolate*
- Navy (haricot) beans and other foods rich in choline
- Pasture-raised meat

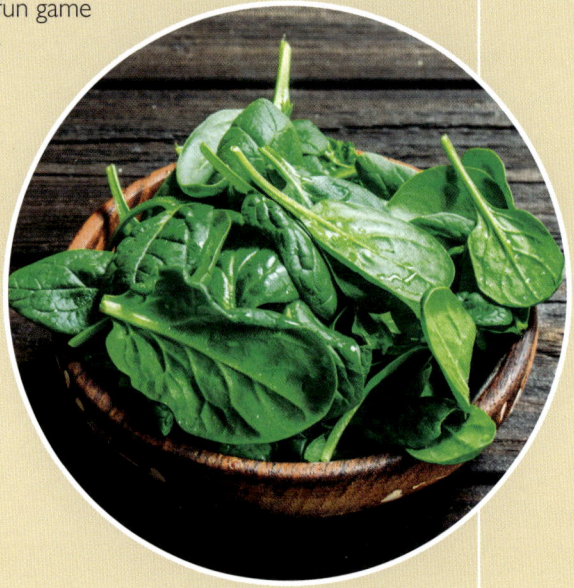

*If you find these starred foods do not improve your energy, mood, and focus, you may be suffering from a sensitivity to them (see page 28).*

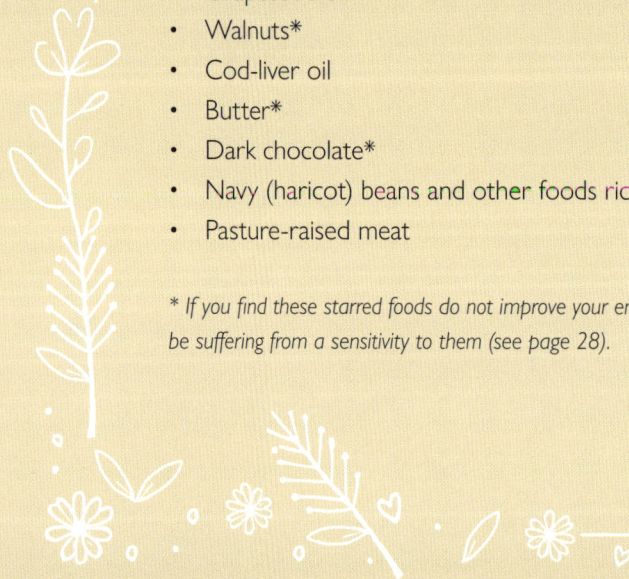

The good news is that there are many healthy options for adding a little sweetness to your day. A serving of mixed berries, pear, banana, and cherries makes a colorful dessert plate that is naturally sweet. On a cold winter day, steamed and puréed yams provide a delicious side dish for your roast turkey. Raw honey, rapadura (unrefined cane sugar), pure maple syrup, and blackstrap molasses can be used instead of refined sugar in traditional baking recipes. Stevia, a natural herbal sweetener, is now a favorite for many (but do avoid it if you have an allergy to ragweed).

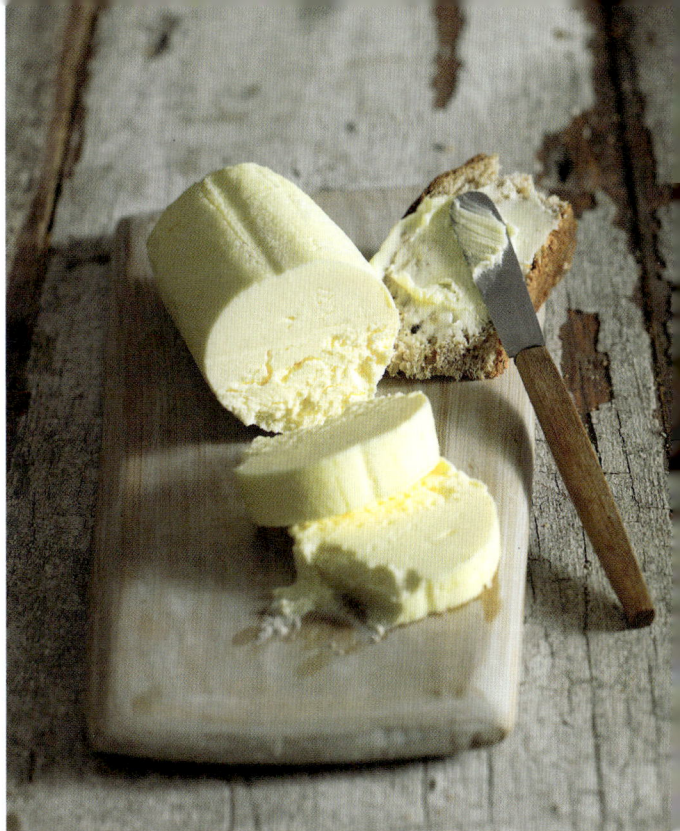

## Cholesterol

Since the 1950s, we have been told that eating saturated fat and cholesterol-rich foods is unhealthy and contributes particularly to heart disease. This was based on flawed studies. Animal fats in foods were said to cause heart disease and cholesterol problems. This was promoted by the vegetable oil industry and conventional medical community, which had strong ties to pharmaceutical industries. Harmful partially hydrogenated processed vegetable oils (including corn, canola, sunflower, cottonseed, and vegetable), margarine and other butter substitutes, and vegetable shortening for baked goods became staples in the food supply.

Thankfully, there is increasing awareness that saturated fat and cholesterol are not the villains in the food supply. With current dietary trends including the Paleo Diet, the Ketogenic Diet, and Whole30®, we are reintegrating traditional fats from responsibly farmed animals into our dietary vocabulary. Gone are the egg-white omelets, margarine, and other artificial butter substitutes; instead butter, duck fat, coconut oil, and lard are slowly making a comeback on the food plate.

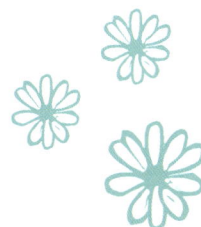

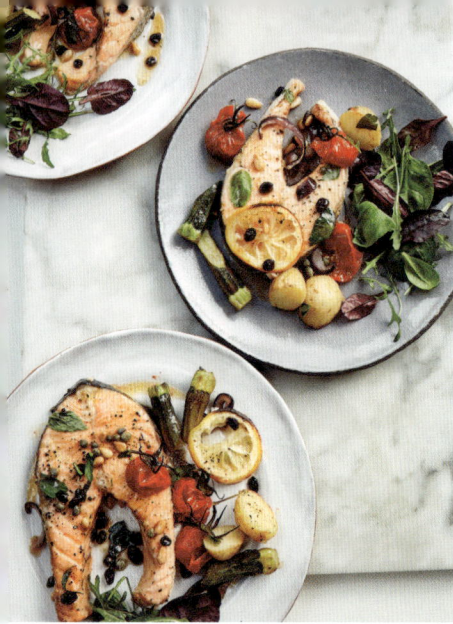

# Managing food sensitivities

No discussion of wellbeing can leave out the implication of the food sensitivities that are so prevalent today, since they greatly affect our energy, mood, and focus.

Food allergies and sensitivities can appear immediately, or as late as 72 hours after the consumption of a food trigger, and symptoms can range from ADHD, itching, swelling, bloating, brain fog, hyper-excitability, seizures, sleepiness, painful joints, headaches, and depression, to life-threatening anaphylaxis, weight gain, and more. There are many reasons why these occur. Common root causes include antibiotics in foods, medication, stress, and gluten, all of which contribute to a leaky gut (see page 20).

Changes to your diet can be very helpful in decreasing the effects. If you suffer from any inflammatory condition, cognitive problems, or mood disorders, consider eliminating gluten to see if it alleviates or even resolves the symptoms. Similarly, eliminate dairy if you have asthma, chronic sinusitis, or ongoing respiratory problems. Why not try eliminating gluten or dairy for three weeks? Note in a food diary how you feel, improvements in your health, and any other changes you observe. After three weeks, have a day full of gluten-containing foods, or multiple glasses of milk, as appropriate. Track how your body responds in the next few days. Food elimination is an inexpensive and effective way of seeing if foods you consume regularly do not agree with you. Your body does not lie. As with all dietary advice in this book, do obtain medical advice from a physician before making changes.

# TOP 14 TRIGGER FOODS

These foods can induce fatigue, headaches, mood swings, and poor concentration. Food allergies and sensitivities can appear immediately, or as late as 72 hours after the consumption of a food trigger.

- Foods containing gluten
- Corn
- Sugar
- Soy
- Foods high in histamine, including spinach, ripe bananas, avocado, and salmon
- Nuts
- Dairy
- Foods high in oxalate, including chocolate, rhubarb, and coffee
- Eggs, especially egg whites
- Artificial sweeteners, which are neurotoxins
- Foods containing yeast
- Alcohol
- Foods high in salicylate, including radishes, strawberries, and wine
- Nightshades, including tomato, eggplant (aubergine), potatoes, and peppers of all kinds

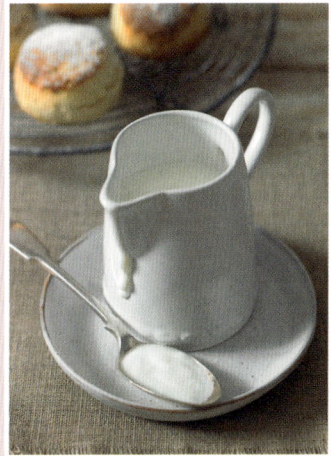

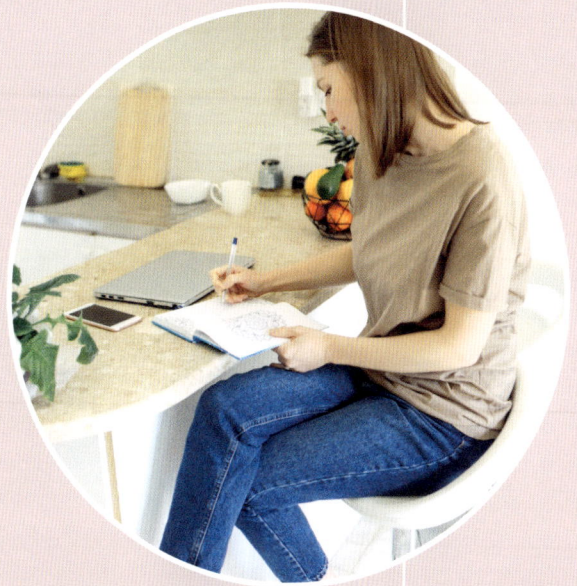

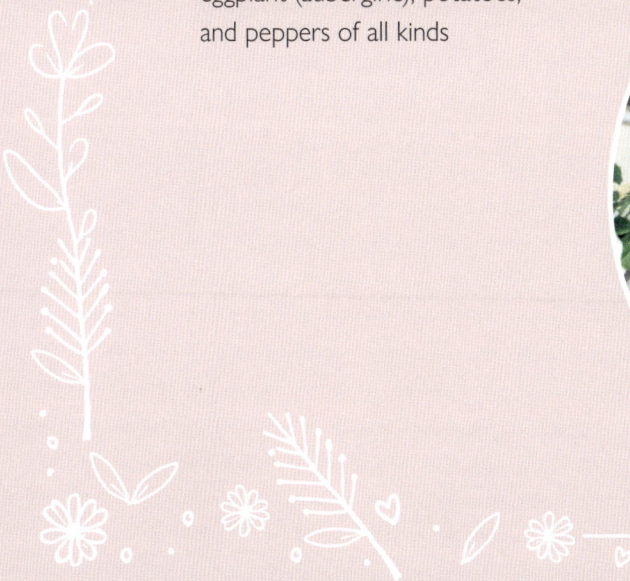

# Prepping your meals for maximum benefit

In today's fast-paced world, the acts of preparing food and cooking at home reconnect us with mindfulness, creativity, and patience.

By preparing and consuming whole foods from the animal and plant kingdoms, we return to our cultural culinary roots. It is at this fundamental level that we create healing opportunities by balancing our gut flora, giving us a greater chance to live a happy life filled with vitality. The quality of the food we use, and how we prepare and cook it, is very important, since it has an impact on how available nutrients are to our bodies.

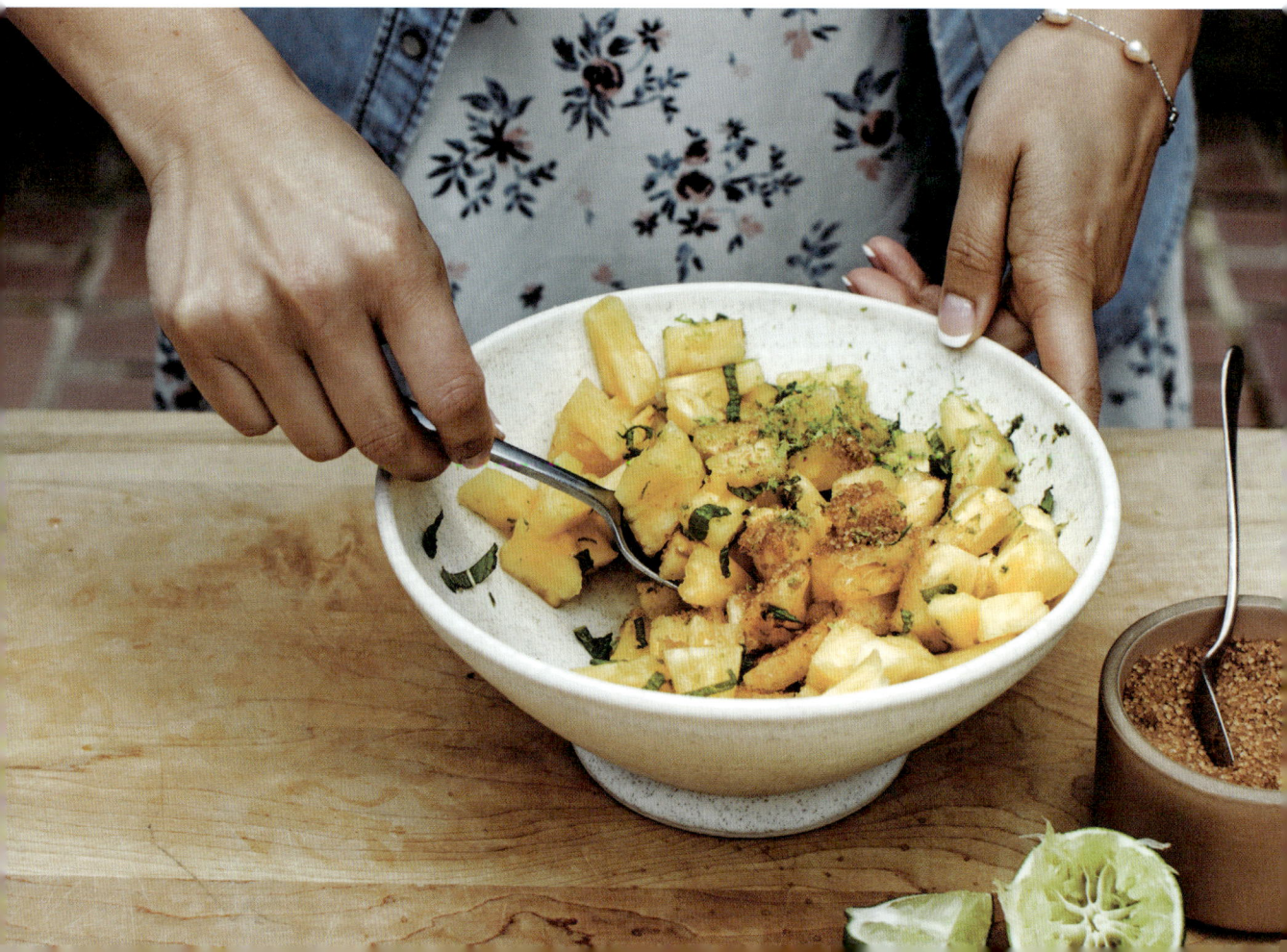

## Meat and fish

Frying, roasting, grilling, and searing protein-rich foods at high temperatures is not recommended, as this destroys nutrients, especially B vitamins. High temperatures produce compounds called advanced glycation end products (AGEs), also called glycotoxins. We absorb these into our bloodstream and they are linked with increased inflammation. This matters when we cook pork, fish, beef, chicken, and eggs, or consume popular steamed drinks with sugary ingredients and artificial flavors. In addition, any browning or blackening of foods, even oozing marshmallows on a stick over a grill or fire, encourages the formation of cancer-causing molecules that can increase inflammation.

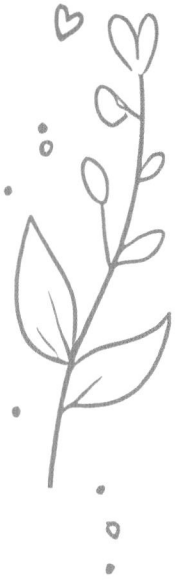

## Fruit and vegetables

When consuming organic lemons and oranges (citrus fruits), integrate the peel. It contains limonene, a potent anti-cancer agent. It is limonene that provides a refreshing aroma and taste. Grate the peel over a salad or add it to your shake to awaken the senses. Pesticides and insecticides are stored in the peel of non-organic fruit and vegetables, so do not consume it even if you wash them well. Chop, slice, squeeze, and dice organic vegetables, fruit, and mushrooms to your heart's delight.

## Grains, nuts, and seeds

Phytic acid, an enzyme inhibitor, is in the fiber of grains, legumes, soybeans, nuts, and seeds. It adversely affects the absorption of B12, iron, and zinc from these foods. However, all these nutrients are needed for thyroid, brain, immune and digestive function. The solution is either to reduce your consumption of these foods, or to consider traditional food preparation methods such as fermentation, germination, and soaking to neutralize phytic acid. This unlocks the nutrients that our body can absorb, but it takes time and effort in the kitchen. (Even corn and rice were fermented in traditional cuisines.) Soak nuts, seeds, or grains overnight in a bowl with either sea salt or apple cider vinegar to get rid of the phytic acid. Grains can be cooked in the morning once you have rinsed them well in a strainer (sieve).

## Fermentation

Fermentation is a traditional method of food preparation that is making a comeback at farmers' markets, restaurants, gourmet stores, and at home. Foods made in this way include the drink known as kombucha, cultured dairy such as kefir, and kimchee. There are various cultured or fermented foods that you can make at home.

## Kitchen equipment

Optimal choices for cooking and baking are:
- Traditional cast-iron cookware, which conducts heat very well, and is durable and good value for money (but avoid using it to cook acidic foods, including tomatoes, which cause the iron to react)
- Copper pots and pans, which also conduct heat very well, but again react with acidic foods
- Ceramic pots for cooking at higher temperatures
- Glass and CorningWare or Pyrex (avoid cheap imitations)
- Stoneware for baking, casseroles, and grilled vegetables
- Stainless steel (although be aware that this can leach nickel during cooking)
- A carbon steel wok
- A cooking thermometer

Invest in sharp knives for meat or poultry, or larger fruit such as melon. Also consider handy 3–4-inch (7.5–10-cm) paring knives for vegetables and fruit, and a serrated bread knife that can also be used for slicing tomatoes, peaches, fatty cuts of meat, and sandwiches for the lunchbox. Use knife-friendly wood or bamboo cutting boards for vegetables and fruit, but for cutting or chopping raw meat, poultry, and seafood, use color-coded plastic boards. All boards can harbor harmful bacteria, so make sure to wash them thoroughly; plastic ones can safely go in the dishwasher. For carving cooked meat, it is great to invest in an additional board; otherwise use the one for vegetables.

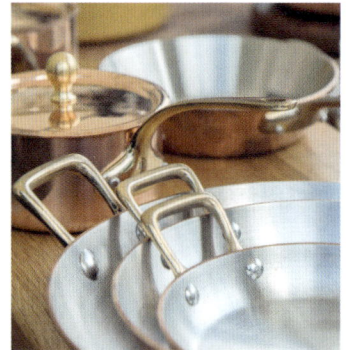

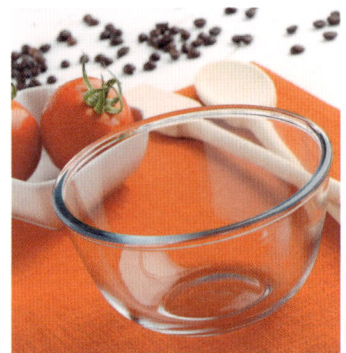

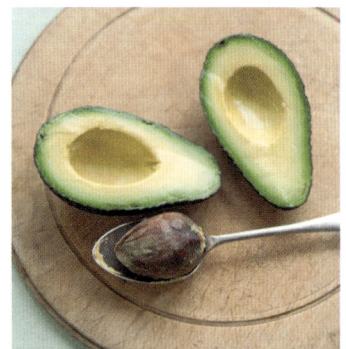

# TOP METHODS FOR HEALTHY FOOD PREP

Food preparation can take time, but it will serve you well over a lifetime. We might think our body doesn't care whether we eat home-prepared meals or store-bought foods, but it does know the difference. Our heart and soul are in the meals we prepare in our own kitchen.

- Braising
- Pan-roasting
- Grilling
- Boiling
- Roasting
- Pan-frying
- Mincing
- Juicing
- Blending
- Raw foods
- Blanching
- Sautéing
- Steaming
- Simmering
- Brining
- Curing
- Poaching
- Baking
- Pickling
- Griddling
- Fermenting
- Slow-cooking
- Stewing
- Canning

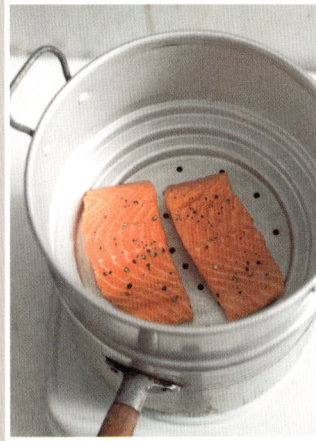

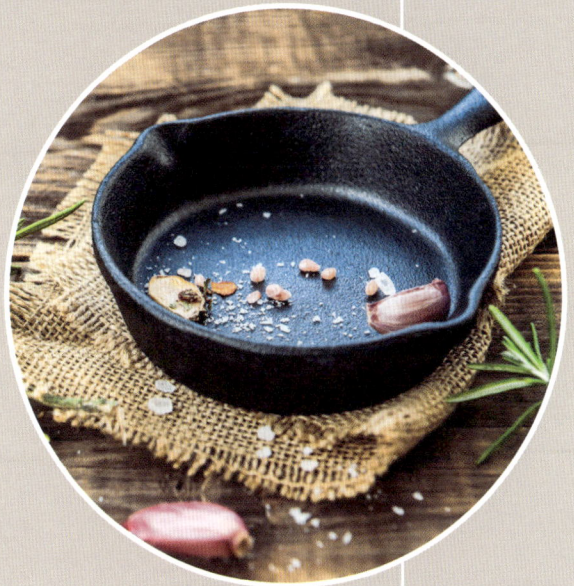

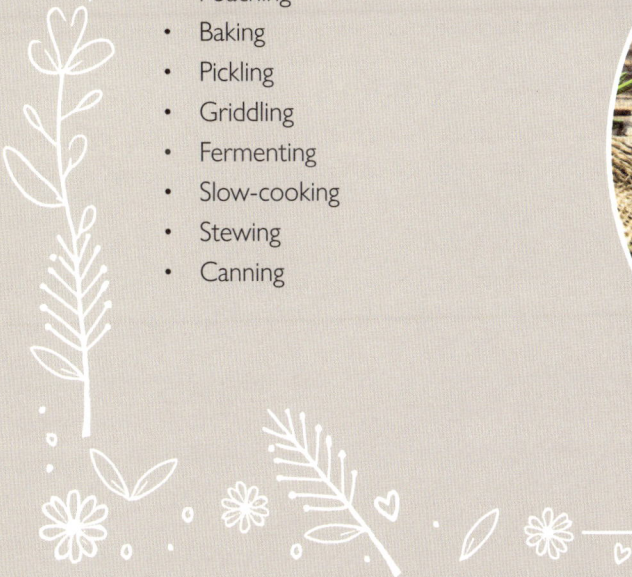

# Slow it down

How you eat is just as important as what you eat. When we pay attention to our experience, we often notice that it changes.

There is a time lag between eating and the brain receiving the message that the stomach is full. When we eat too quickly or are distracted, we don't create the opportunity to receive this message. However, when we take our time, we notice when the body says "enough," and because we are aware of the experience, the food seems much more fulfilling than usual. Therefore, when we eat mindfully, we usually eat less because we are listening to the body.

Mindful eating is best done in silence, although you can do it with others if they remain silent, too. Maintaining silence in this practice reminds us that we are doing something differently—in this case, that we are eating a meal in a way we usually don't. Silence is often like an "on" switch. Without the interruptions of talking and listening, we naturally pay attention to what we are eating, and as we pay attention we slow down accordingly. We notice how the body reacts in anticipation of the next spoonful. We chew our food rather than swallow it automatically. Perhaps we feel the stomach expanding and becoming fuller with every mouthful. We pause between mouthfuls. We are aware of the crunchy texture of this carrot; the juiciness of that tomato; the delicate flavor of this spice, the strong taste of that herb. We become aware of what we are eating.

As we become aware of what we are putting into our mouths, we begin to make deliberate choices. If we are focusing on tasting our food, we want it to taste as good as it can be. We begin noticing how we feel after certain foods and naturally gravitate toward those that give us energy rather than make us feel sluggish. Also, we become aware of the point of choice when we are reaching for something—this gives us time to pause and make a conscious decision about what we are going to eat, rather than eating mindlessly.

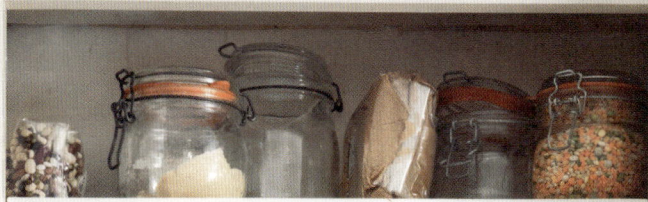

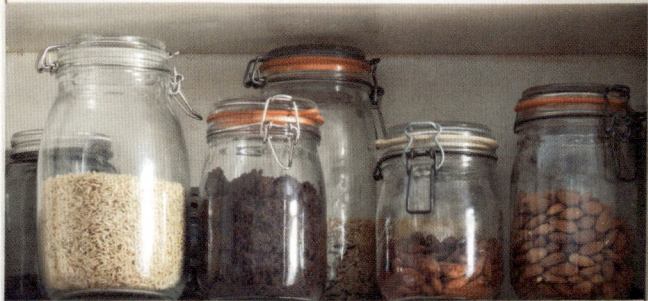

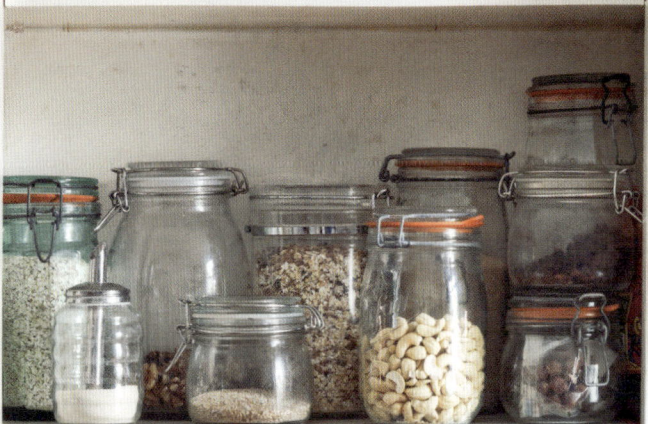

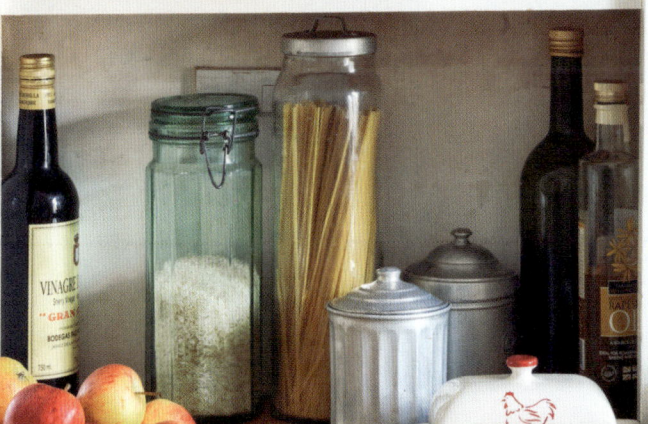

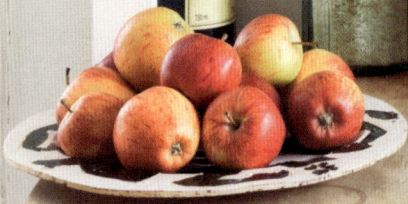

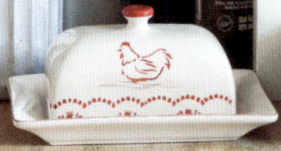

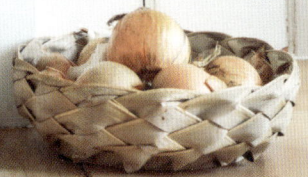

# Rotate your plate

We need to eat a variety of natural compounds known as phytonutrients, polyphenols, flavonoids, ellagic acid, and carotenoids found in plant-based foods if our mind and body are to be well.

Thankfully, nature provides us with an abundance of fruit and vegetables that delight the eye, nose, and palate. Every food contains a different array of vitamins, minerals, and fiber that interacts with our unique biochemistry.

It is important to respect the climate we live in when we make our daily food choices. In colder climates or chilly weather, choose warming oatmeal (porridge), hearty soups, stews, and curries of all kinds. In sunny and warm climates or seasons, smoothies, crisp, light salads, and chilled soups help to cool the body. Availability is another important consideration: If you live in Northern Europe, for example, where the winters are rainy and gray, you may have a more limited choice of local fresh fruit and vegetables at certain times than do those who live in sunshine-filled Florida.

Food rotation is not a novel concept, nor is the emphasis on eating seasonal and local foods. Be aware that any long-term food elimination or dietary strategy that eliminates a macronutrient (such as the vegan diet, which contains no animal proteins or fats) may cause nutrient deficiencies over time. Depending on where you live, different foods will be available to you, and by eating a kaleidoscope of local fruits, medicinal mushrooms, and seasonal vegetables, you can incorporate their innate healing properties into your body.

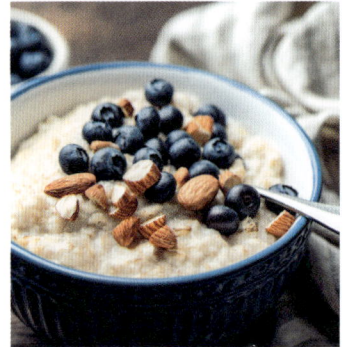

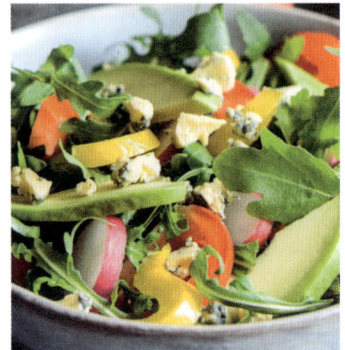

# Nourishing your chakras

Foods matter on an energetic level; after all, food = energy. Every color of the rainbow connects to one of the seven energetic points in our body, known as chakras. Through mindful choices of diet, we can nourish our emotional wellness, too.

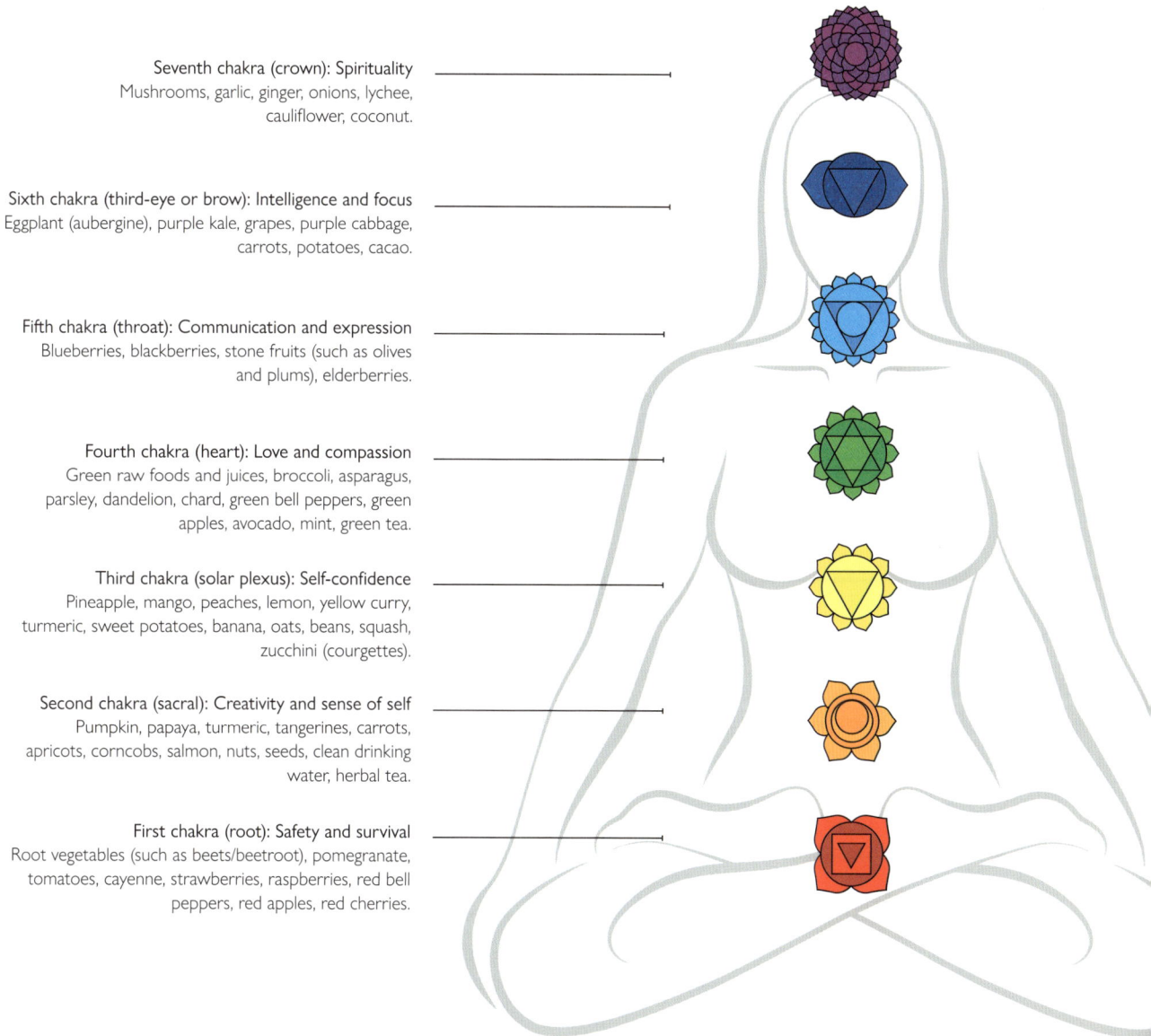

**Seventh chakra (crown): Spirituality**
Mushrooms, garlic, ginger, onions, lychee, cauliflower, coconut.

**Sixth chakra (third-eye or brow): Intelligence and focus**
Eggplant (aubergine), purple kale, grapes, purple cabbage, carrots, potatoes, cacao.

**Fifth chakra (throat): Communication and expression**
Blueberries, blackberries, stone fruits (such as olives and plums), elderberries.

**Fourth chakra (heart): Love and compassion**
Green raw foods and juices, broccoli, asparagus, parsley, dandelion, chard, green bell peppers, green apples, avocado, mint, green tea.

**Third chakra (solar plexus): Self-confidence**
Pineapple, mango, peaches, lemon, yellow curry, turmeric, sweet potatoes, banana, oats, beans, squash, zucchini (courgettes).

**Second chakra (sacral): Creativity and sense of self**
Pumpkin, papaya, turmeric, tangerines, carrots, apricots, corncobs, salmon, nuts, seeds, clean drinking water, herbal tea.

**First chakra (root): Safety and survival**
Root vegetables (such as beets/beetroot), pomegranate, tomatoes, cayenne, strawberries, raspberries, red bell peppers, red apples, red cherries.

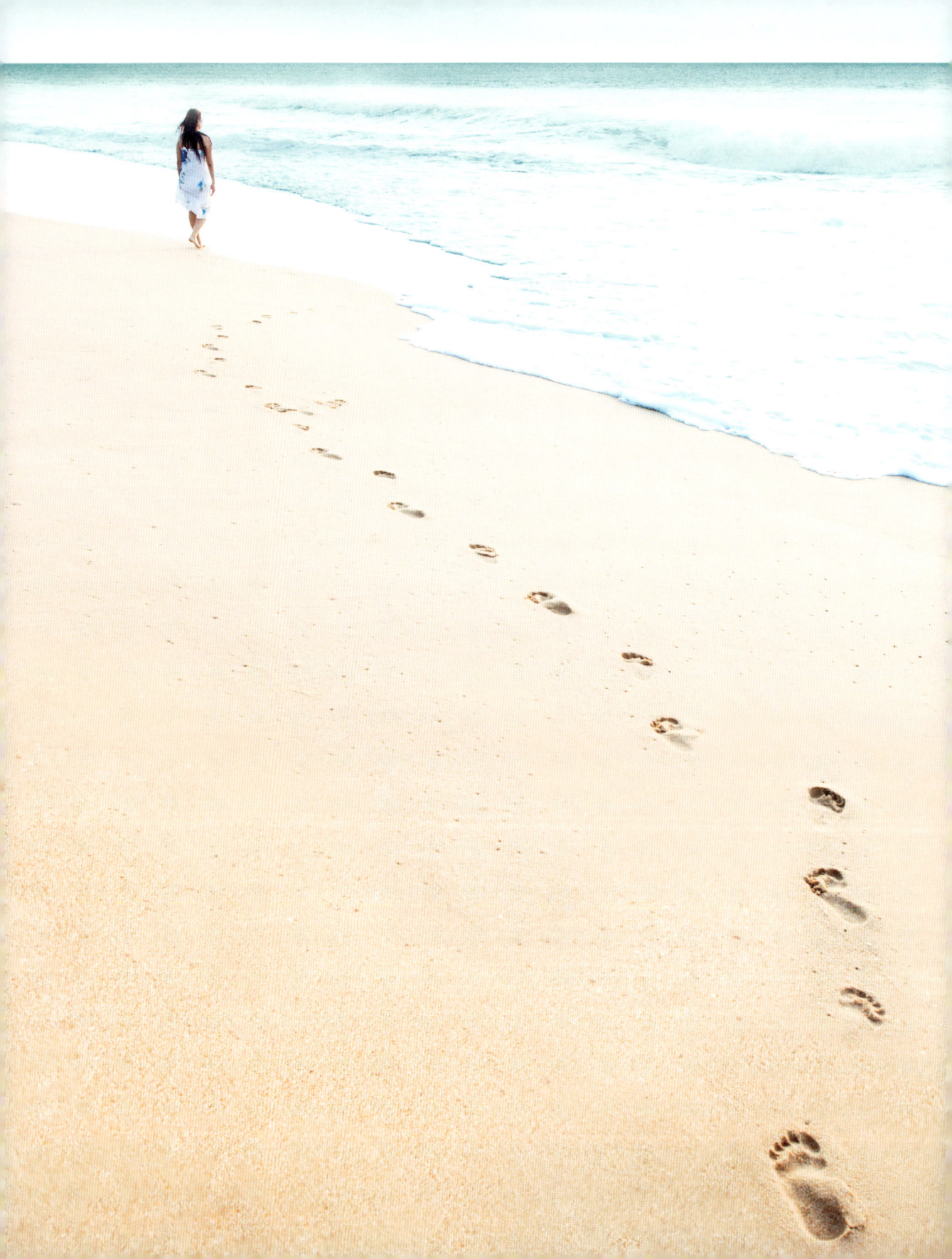

# Chapter 2

# Mindful
# *Movement*

Discover how gentle exercises can refresh your
energy, enhance your overall wellbeing,
and address specific physical and
emotional challenges.

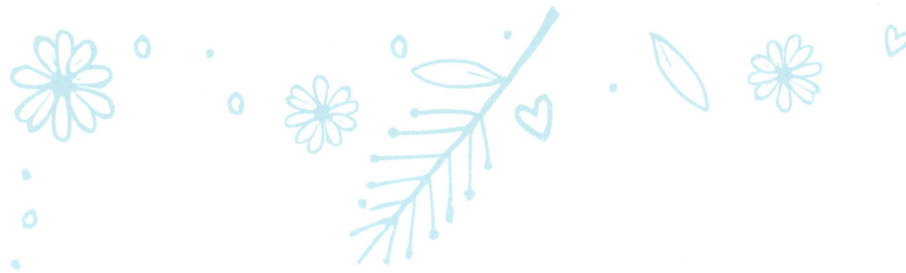

# The importance of movement

It's difficult to stay active and move your body daily when you are busy taking care of kids, working long hours at a desk, spending time with family, or just trying to do it all.

However, movement is vital for your health (not just your physical health but also your mental health). If we are feeling stressed, a brisk walk, run, or swim can help disperse stress hormones such as adrenaline, which can keep us in a state of arousal. Exercise tones your body, keeps you healthy, and boosts your mood, which in turn helps self-esteem and self-confidence. And let's face it, when we feel good about ourselves, we feel happier, too, which leads to a positive frame of mind. So instead of looking at movement—whether it be yoga, the gym, sports, dance, classes, etc—as a chore, try thinking about moving your body as a form of self-love. The more we love ourselves, the more we thrive.

Every day you have an opportunity to honor your body by nourishing it, moving it, and loving it. When you stay active and keep your body moving in an organic way that is a natural complement to the energetics of your body, you will find that life flows with more ease and less stress. Movement is a huge part of longevity and living a balanced life. When you move your body you are treating yourself with the respect you deserve. Your body deserves to be treated right 100 percent of the time. You may find it difficult to stay motivated when it comes to daily movement, but doing at least ten minutes of designated yoga (see pages 54–69) or any other activity will really help your mind–body connection and create more space for healing.

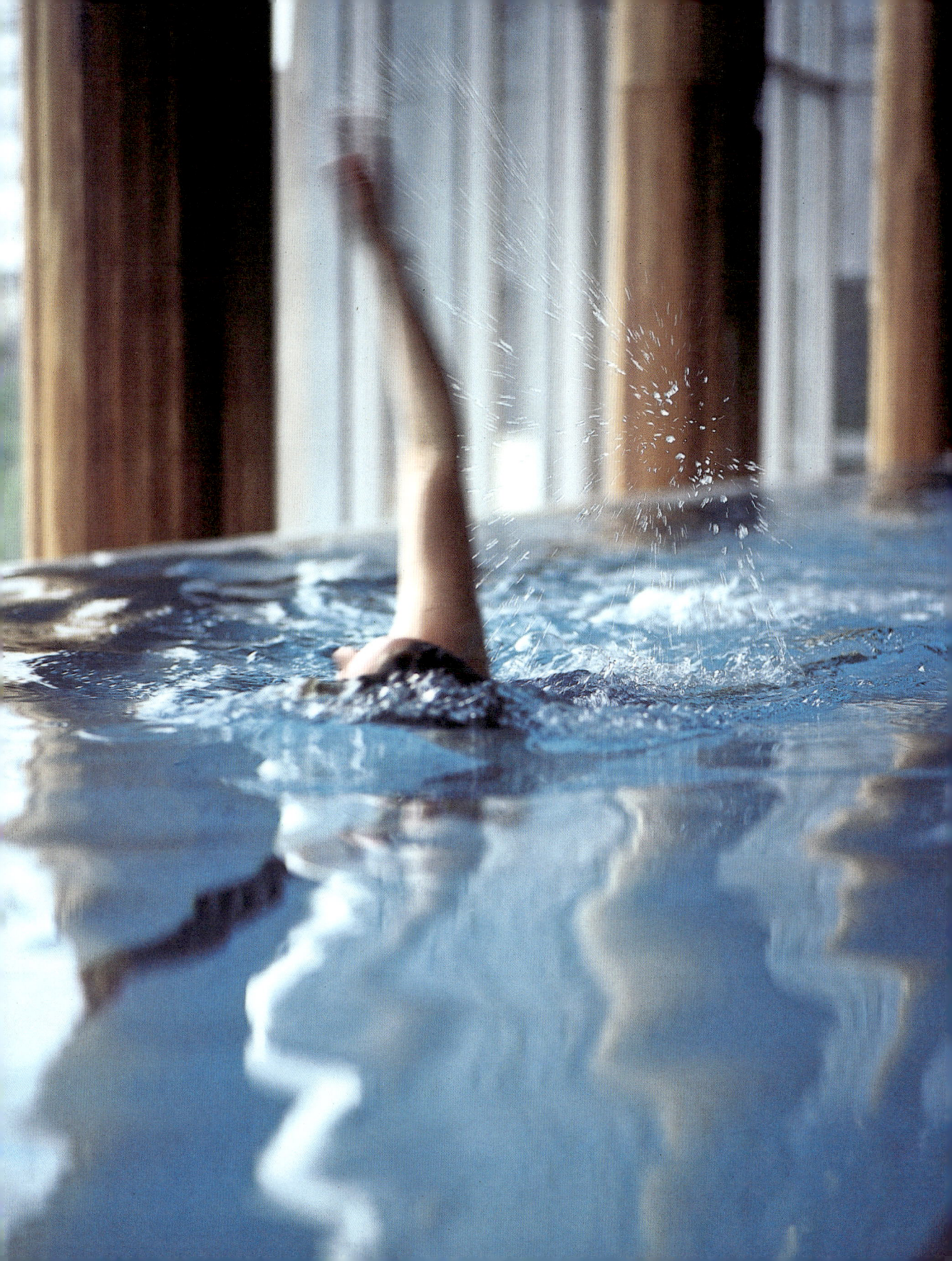

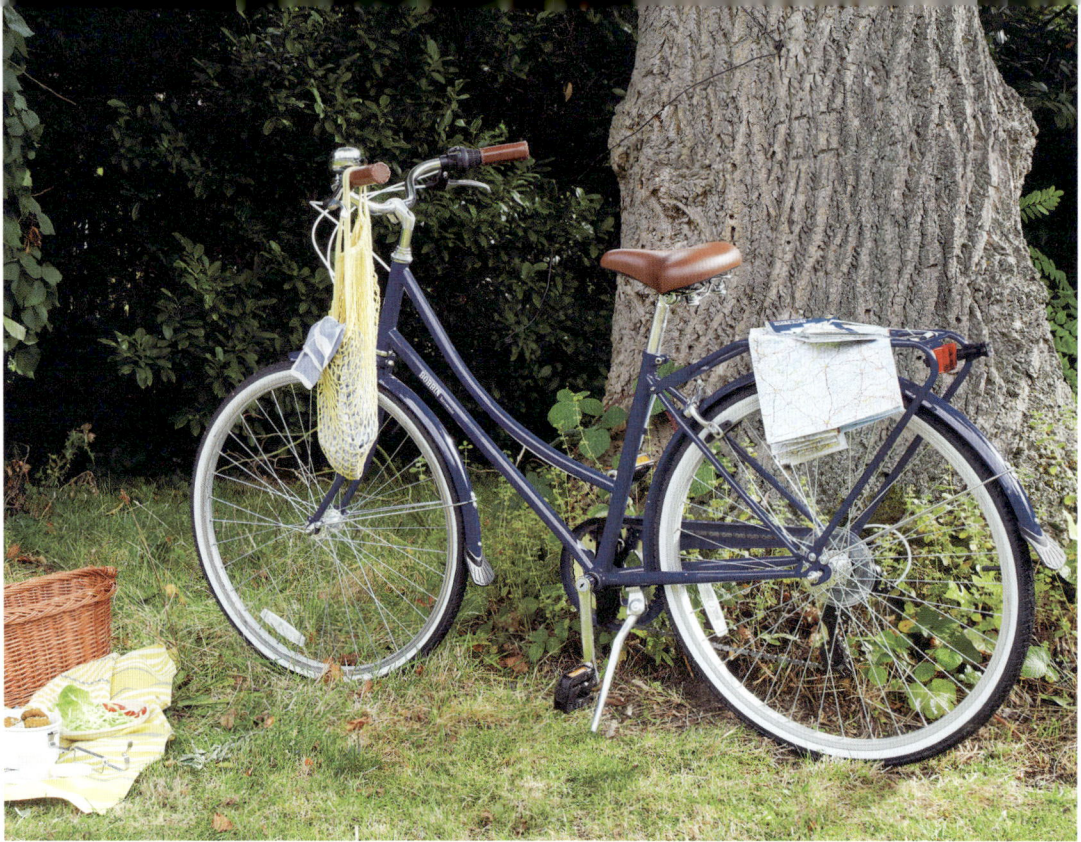

## Changing your attitude

The Cochrane Review is the most influential review of its kind in the world. It has produced an analysis of 23 studies on exercise and depression. Their results showed unequivocally the impact that exercise has on lowering the incidence of depression. Exercise was shown to be as effective as antidepressant medication in helping to reduce mental symptoms. Controversy remains about whether exercise leads to improved mental wellbeing, or whether those with positive mental wellbeing are more likely to exercise—but for anyone non-medical, the message is the same: Exercise makes you happier.

Science tells us that those people who exercise at least two or three times per week experience significantly less depression, anger, and stress than those who exercise less frequently or not at all. If you are feeling a bit low, a quick 20-minute burst of exercise can change your mood and raise your happiness levels. Those who do battle with depression are encouraged to exercise for 30 minutes per day for a minimum of three to five days each week.

## A VARIETY OF BENEFITS

Exercise can help you achieve many different goals:

- "I want to feel calmer and happier." If you are feeling uptight or angry, exercise will help to release tension.
- "I feel overwhelmed by my problems." Many people, including business leaders and politicians, go walking or running when they have to think through a problem.
- "I want to lose weight and look great." Many people lose weight through exercise rather than going on a diet.
- "I want to look younger." Exercise keeps the blood healthy and helps the skin to renew and replenish old cells. It will help you sleep better, too, all of which adds up to a more youthful and energetic you.

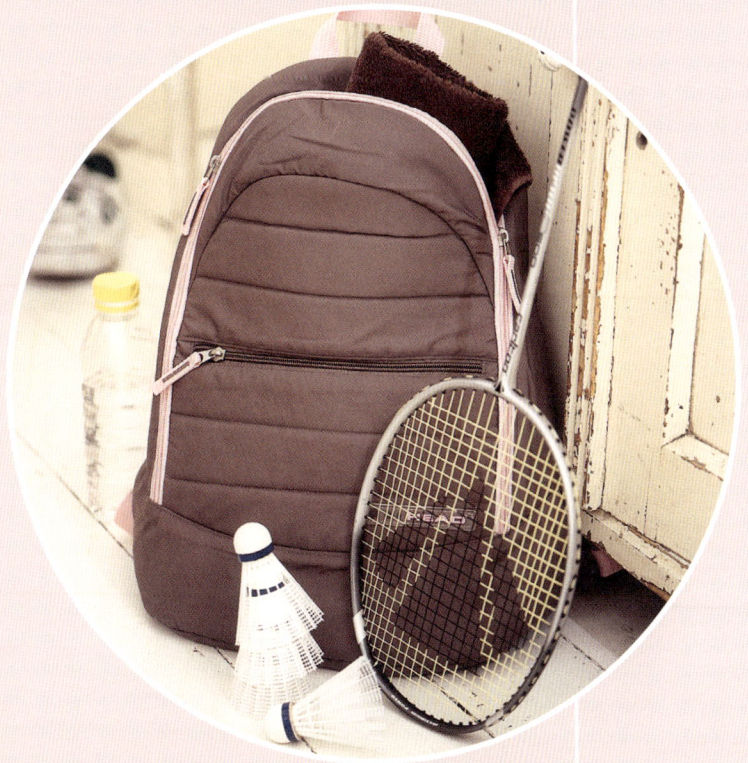

# Do what you can

The world tends to be divided between those who love to exercise—and those who prefer to talk about why they should exercise.

When you are starting out with exercise, short-term goals that include the "happy factor" are more motivating than long-term goals. For example, telling yourself, "It's a beautiful day for a walk and the fresh air will clear my head," is more motivating than "I must go for a run around the block, it will lower my cholesterol".

Think about and write down what exercises and movement you already do. This might include walking to the store or with the children to school, or perhaps you are on your feet all day at home or at work. Include any form of movement that you do in your day. You might do more than you think. (See page 46 for inspiration.)

However, if you find that you do very little exercise or if you would simply like to do more, start to think about what you could do. What is stopping you? Notice any thoughts that arise. Explore the resistance if it feels particularly strong. It is always better to start small and build up your capacity gradually—just adding a few extra steps a day can set you on the right path. Digital trackers that count steps and other activity can be a good incentive. Exercising outside has the added benefit of allowing you to get a dose of fresh air and connect with the natural world (see page 48).

Many activities can be adapted if you have limited mobility (yoga, as featured on pages 54–69, is a particularly good example), but always discuss your needs with an experienced practitioner. It's important that any exercise is suitable for your age and health. If you haven't exercised for a while and you have health problems, do consult your physician first.

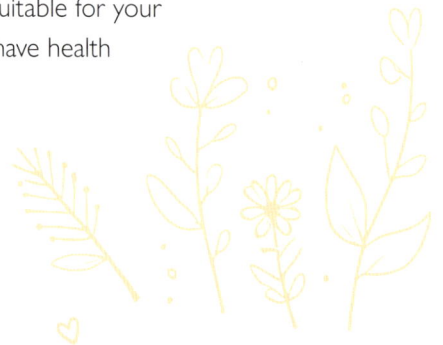

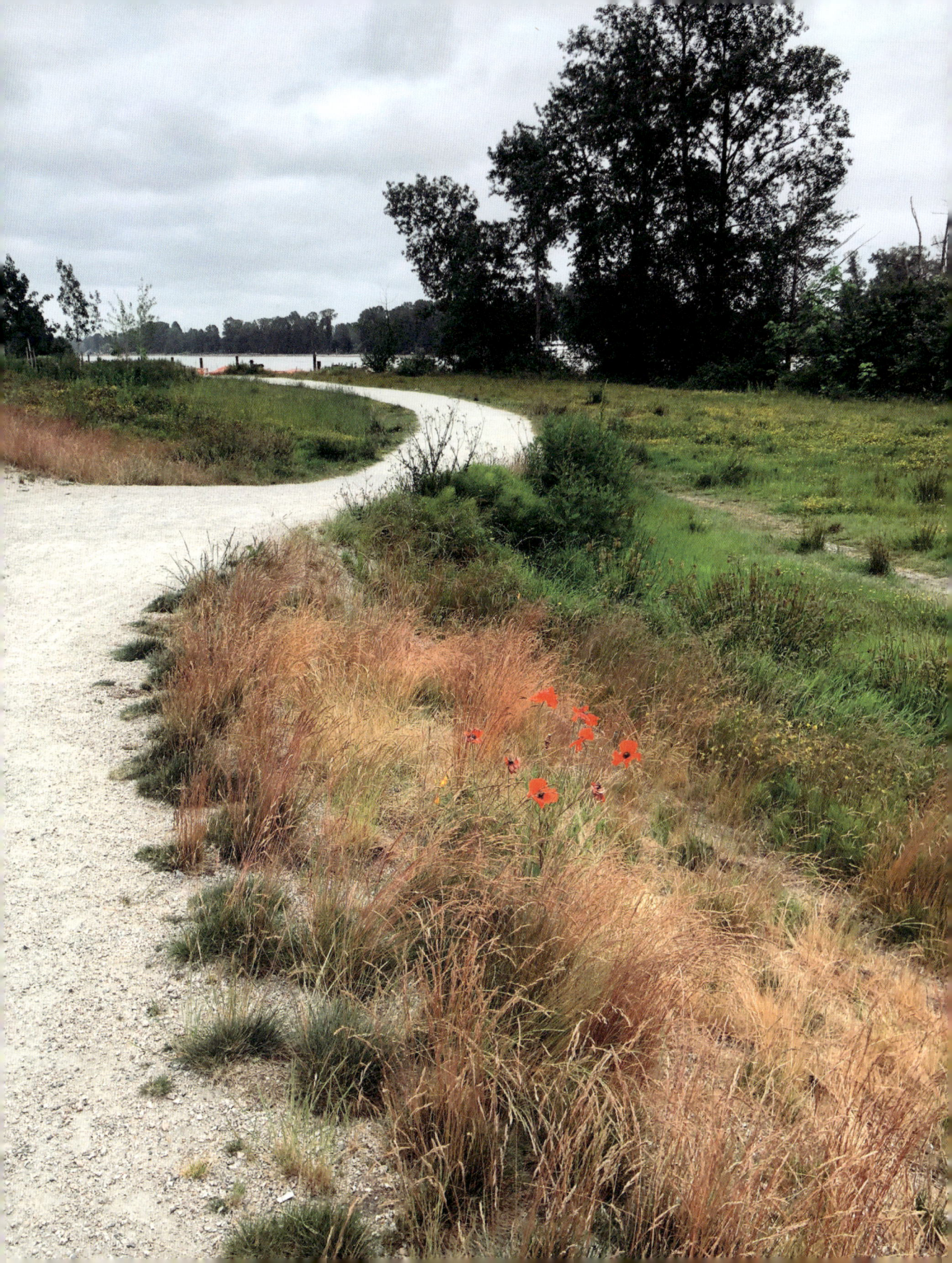

# EASY WAYS TO GET MOVING

Movement can be done anywhere, at any time, and every little bit you do counts! Here are five ways to stay active:

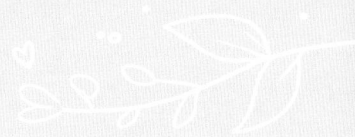

**Stretch, dance, jump around, and move as soon as you wake up in the morning:** Five minutes is all you need. This not only gets your energy up for the day but also wakes up all your body parts.

**Walk or bike to work:** Doing some movement before you start work will increase your focus and prolong your energy. If your work is too far away to walk or bike, park your car farther away from your place of work and walk the longest distance possible to get there.

**Stop, drop, and stretch:** Try to take a two-minute break from work every hour to move your body in an organic way. This will help you feel motivated and ready to work again. You don't only have to stretch, you could do push-ups, crunches, squats, planks, dance, whatever feels right to you.

**Take a break:** Whether you work from home or elsewhere, you can add movement into your post-lunchtime routine. Light movement, like walking, is helpful for digestion after you have eaten. Either walk to a park to eat your lunch and then walk back, or take a walk around the block after you eat. If you live in a very cold climate and work in an office, just take a walk up and down the stairs if you don't want to go outdoors.

**Do activities with friends:** It's much easier to stay motivated when you have a partner to help keep you accountable. Suggest going for a walk instead of meeting for tea to chat. Instead of going out to a bar, go to a salsa or Zumba class and shake your hips. There are plenty of fun activities you can do with others that will keep you connected while moving together.

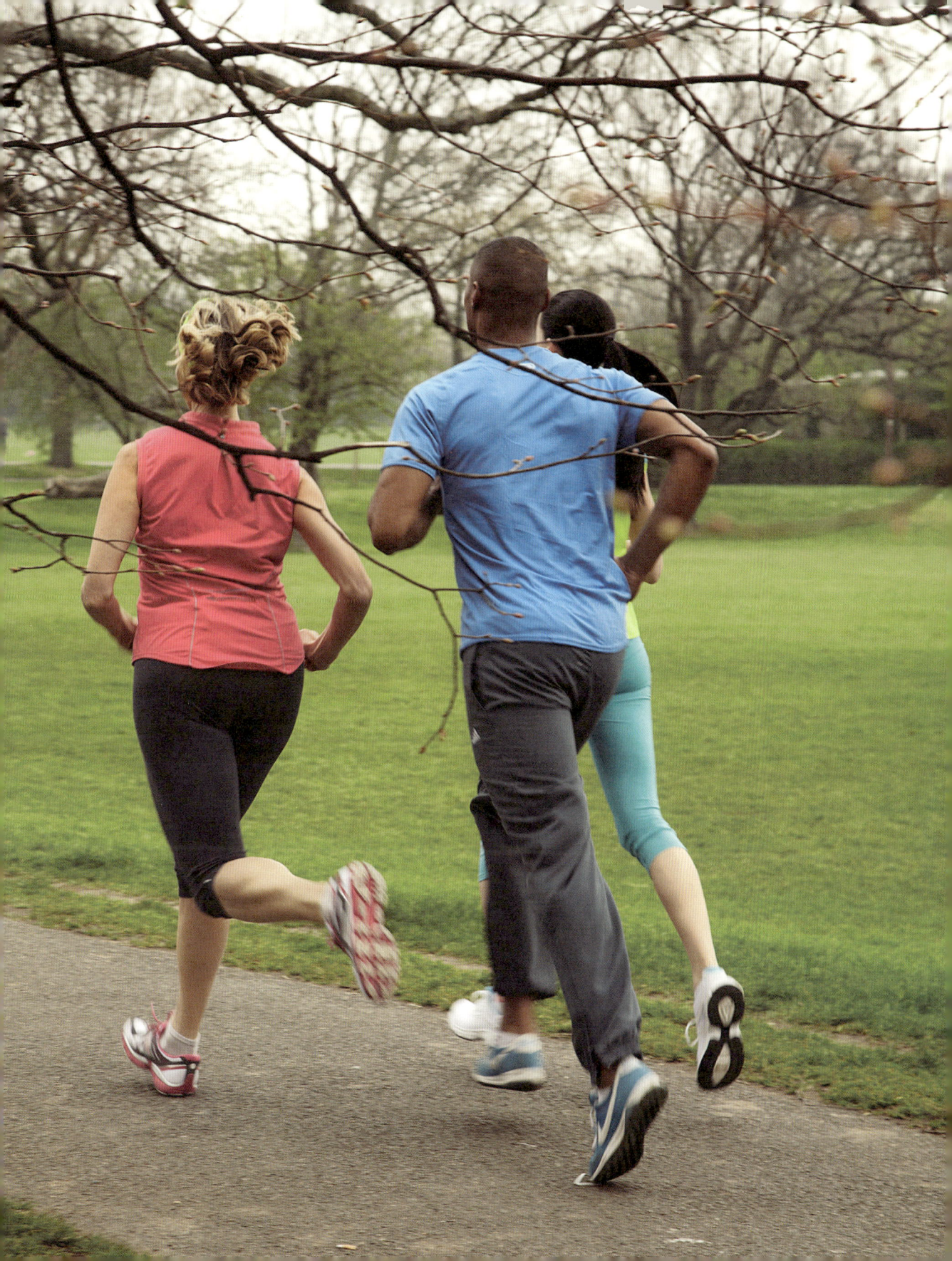

# Take your movement outside

As we've already said, any kind of movement is good for you, but movement outdoors is particularly beneficial. You will get even more vitamin D—the sunshine vitamin—from that than from working out near an open window.

You will also experience a better physical and mental workout navigating uneven outdoor terrain rather than the consistent surface of a treadmill. Plus, you will be able to greet and maybe get to know other walkers, thereby connecting with people and building community, and you can do your own small part for the environment by picking up a bit of trash to improve the aesthetics of your route.

Poets, painters, scientists, and efficiency experts have all commented on how time in nature works as a balm for our minds and a way to de-stress. Former competitive racewalker and cancer survivor Carolyn Scott Kortge supports this idea in her book *Healing Walks for Hard Times: Quiet Your Mind, Strengthen Your Body, and Get Your Life Back* (2010). She reveals how taking a walk is about far more than exercise; it can serve as "a form of stress release and healing that supports medical treatment and emotional recovery." The basic ambulatory act increases our exhalations and inhalations, causing us to release endorphins—from the term "endogenous morphine"—that trigger a natural opioid effect, making us feel happier and more optimistic, while decreasing our perception of pain. It's those hormones that cause the well-known "runner's high."

Numerous studies have shown that walking encourages the front region of our brain—the hypothalamus, which controls temperature, thirst, and hunger, and affects sleep and emotions—to manufacture oxytocin, often known as the love hormone. This acts as a neurotransmitter in the brain, stimulating feelings of empathy and affection. And with love often comes happiness. Walking can make us more joyful. A series of studies by the University of Michigan have shown that this is true no matter one's age—from schoolchildren to the elderly.

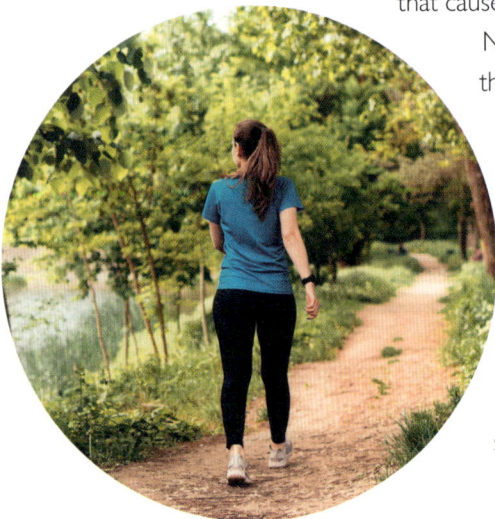

These benefits to our health have to do with overriding rumination—our tendency to dwell on troubling thoughts or worry about everything from finances to our child's hurt feelings. Long-term rumination, marked by activity in the part of the brain that controls emotions and the personality (the prefrontal cortex), can lead to depression, but walking in nature has been shown to decrease rumination. A Stanford University study found that taking a 90-minute walk through a natural environment as opposed to an urban one reduces rumination and consequently the neural activity in the part of the brain that is linked to the risk of mental illness.

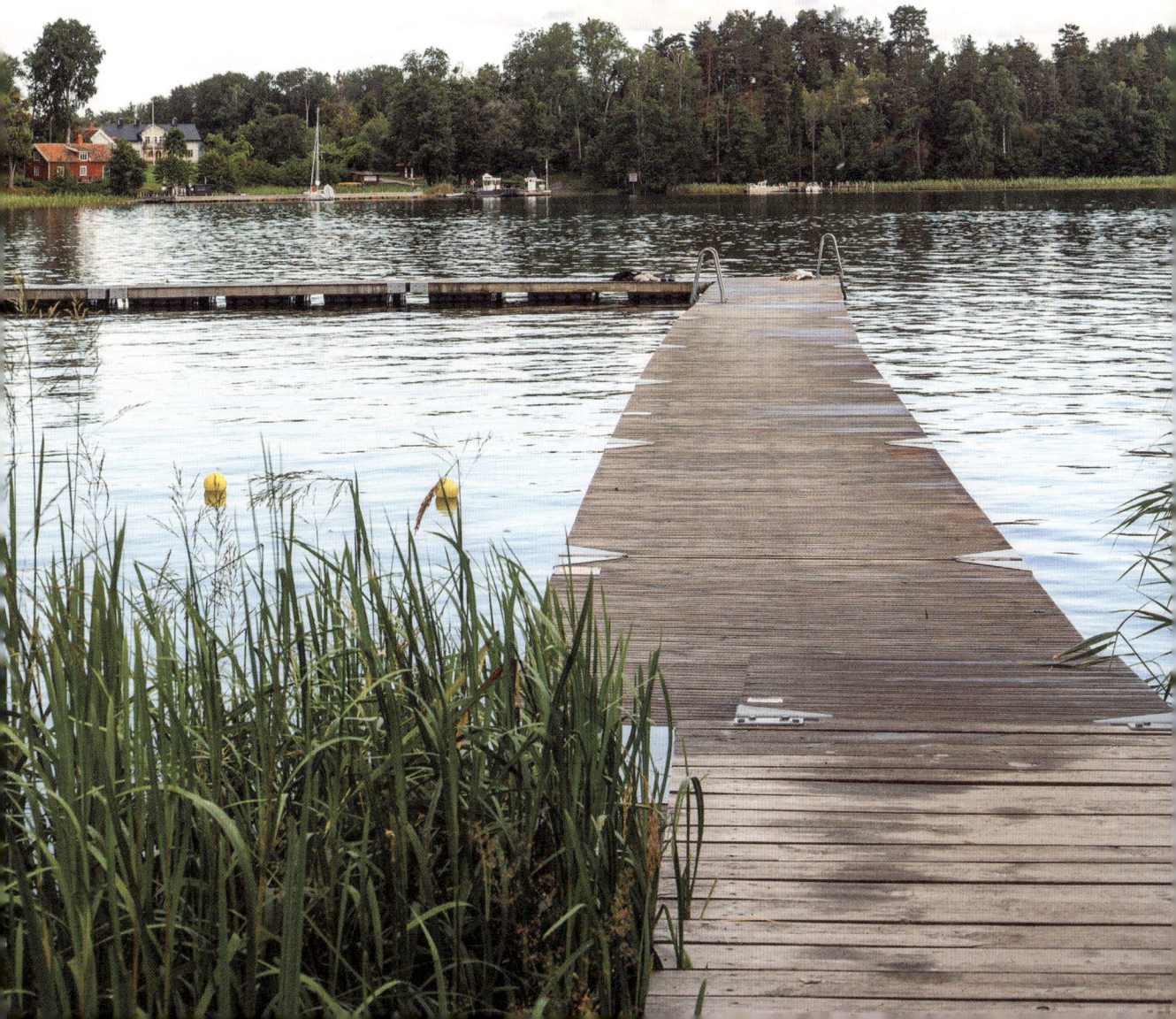

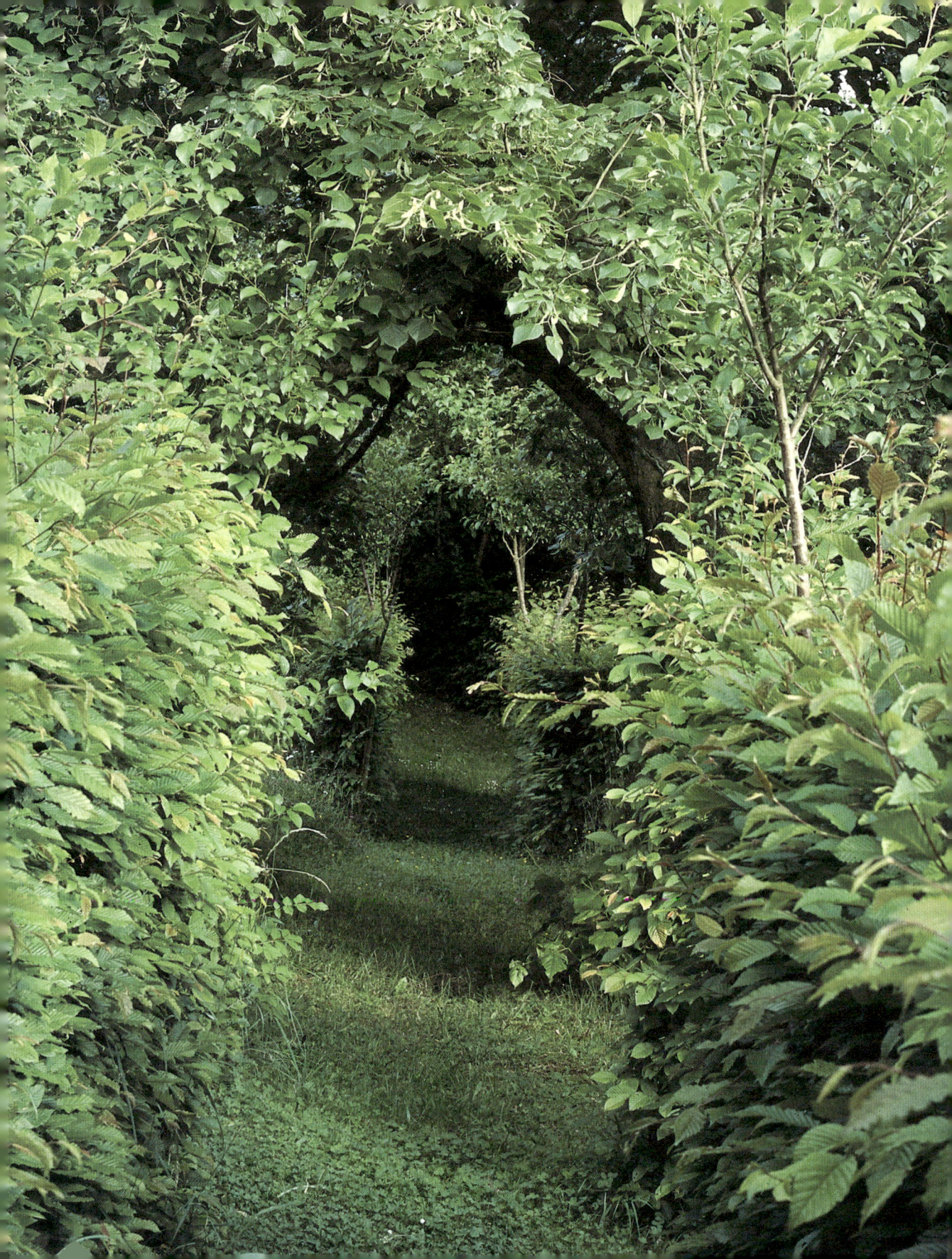

# Boost your workout with forest bathing

Any walk outdoors is good for you, but if you can get to some woods, that's even better. Over the past few years, more people have become intrigued by the concept of forest bathing—healing through the contemplative practice of intentionally spending time with trees—and it has really caught on. Forest bathing is being taught and practiced at botanic gardens, spas, spiritual retreats, and recreation centers. Beyond that, it is being used in psychiatric hospitals, in conjunction with physical therapy, and in addiction treatment programs.

In 1982, Tomohide Akiyama, then secretary of Japan's Ministry of Agriculture, Forestry, and Fisheries, coined the term "shinrin-yoku." This translates as "forest bathing," and can be defined as making contact with and being affected—both physically and mentally—by the atmosphere of the forest. Perhaps more aptly called "forest basking," since neither soap nor tub is involved, forest bathing can be experienced as a type of meditation, and, just as with other Eastern-rooted practices such as mindfulness, Ayurvedic medicine, and yoga, Westerners are learning that there is far more to meditation than simply becoming calm. Many authorities are in agreement that meditation can ease psychological problems from anxiety to post-traumatic stress disorder, help to treat addiction, make us better parents and workers, and promote the healing of many physical ailments.

Forest bathing incorporates many of the benefits of meditation while getting us outdoors and in motion. In a study conducted by the College of Landscape Architecture at Sichuan Agricultural University, Chengdu, China, 30 men and 30 women were given a route of the same length to walk in either a bamboo forest or an urban area. The results showed that, although walking is good for you, walking among trees is much better. The researchers measured blood pressure as well as electrical activity in the brain using an EEG (electroencephalogram), and they found that, among those who walked the forest path, blood pressure was lowered significantly as attention and concentration improved. The people walking in nature reported less anxiety and a generally happier mood than the urban group.

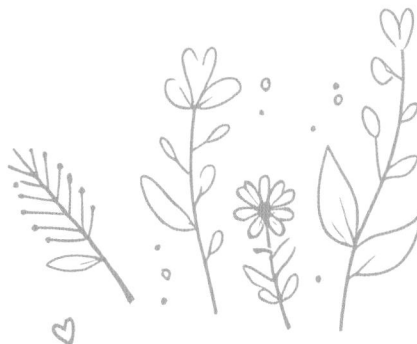

# How to breathe better

It seems pretty obvious to say that we need to breathe in order to live, but did you know you can use your breath to maximize your lifespan, combat stress, and manipulate the energetic flow in your body? Plus, when combined with exercise, it maximizes the benefits.

The Sanskrit word *prana* means both "life-force energy" and "breath;" it doesn't have a single direct translation or function. According to Ayurveda (a traditional Indian system of medicine), prana is considered the root source of all the energy in the universe. All forces of nature are manifestations of prana. Think about your breath as a subtle force that not only fills your physical body with life-giving energetic oxygen but also fills your mind and emotional body with energetic vitality. When we inhale both deeply and consciously, we breathe oxygen into our lungs as well as take in the environment and knowledge found in all of life.

Prana is the driving force behind all things. It is prana that keeps things moving in and around us. Without prana, life is gray, dark, cloudy, and full of stagnant energy. With prana, life is bright, creative, open, full, loving, and flowing. Prana can be found in the food we eat, the liquid we drink, the air we breathe, the warmth of the sun, and the people and places around us. This is why relationships feel so good—we are transferring this pranic energy from person to person. Likewise, illness and symptoms of sickness are clear manifestations of obstructed or decreased pranic flow.

Whether you subscribe to this belief or not, breathing exercises really can be effective for reducing stress and anxiety, improving lung function, and promoting relaxation.

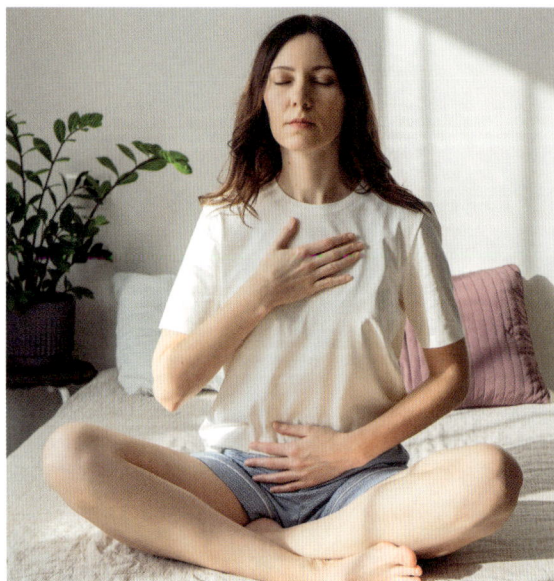

## SIMPLE BREATHING EXERCISE

This exercise is called a pranic breath, and it's great at releasing stress. Start with one pranic breath and work your way up (in your own time) to ten. Do this practice at least once a day.

- Sit comfortably, cross-legged on the floor, if possible. You can use a bolster or blankets to prop your legs up or lean against a wall to help you sit up tall. Try to relax your shoulders, allowing your shoulder blades to roll down your back toward your waist. This will help to lift your chest up and create space for your ribcage to move freely.
- Place your palms together in front of your heart. Push with pressure against both palms to create an activation of energy between both spheres of the body.
- Gently close your lips and focus only on breathing through your nose.
- Inhale for the count of ten, breathing in deeply through your nose and drawing your breath down into your lungs. Feel the breath expanding in your ribcage and trickling down into your belly, expanding deeper and wider. Imagine this breath as a golden white light that is pulling in all of Mother Nature's beautiful invigorating energy and sucking it deep into your body.
- Once your lungs and belly are full of this life-giving air, hold your breath for the count of ten (or as long as possible). Focus all of this energy to your third eye (the middle point in between your eyebrows). Imagine this space filling with all the golden white light that is building and swirling with prana.
- Exhale for the count of ten. As you slowly exhale, imagine the golden white light showering over your whole body and leaving you energized and with all your senses vital.

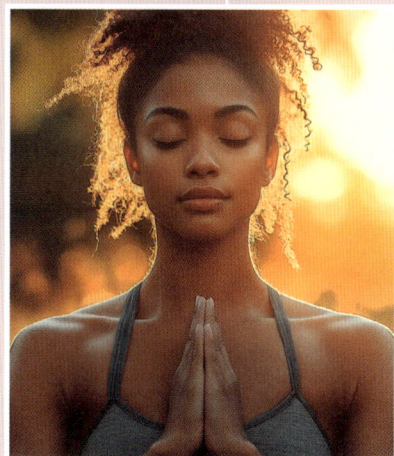

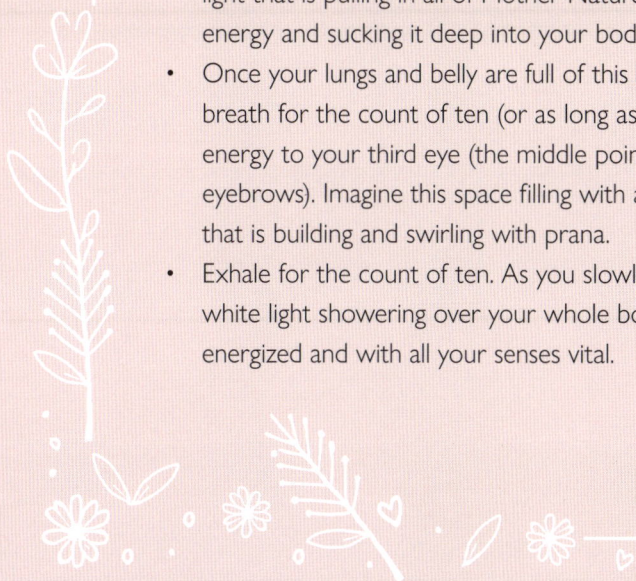

# Yoga poses for anywhere

Yoga is a popular exercise choice because it offers a blend of physical and mental benefits, and can be adapted to various fitness levels. It improves flexibility, strength, and balance while also promoting relaxation and stress reduction. The low-impact nature of yoga makes it accessible to a wide range of individuals, including those new to exercise.

Here are a few yoga poses (asanas) you can do anywhere, anytime. These simple practices can release stress, improve mobility, promote healthy circulation throughout the body, open up energy in the lower spine, massage internal organs, and aid digestion. Remember to practice your pranic breath (see page 53) while trying them.

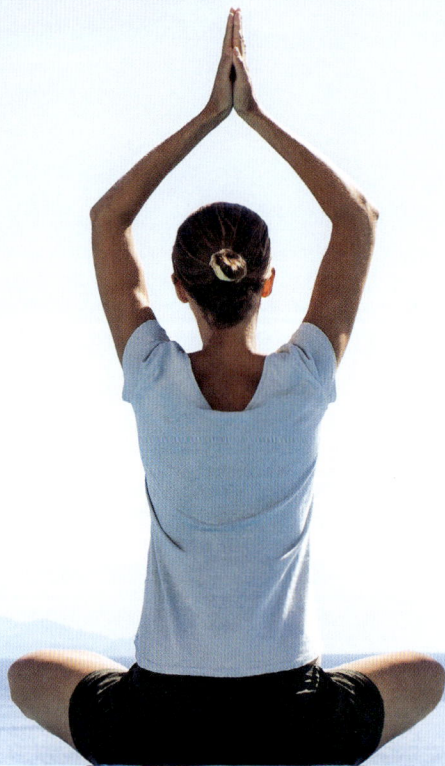

## Spinal Flex

This pose is great for anyone who does little-to-no movement during their day, particularly those who are stuck behind a desk or who spend all their time driving around in a car. You don't even have to get up! You may do the Spinal Flex as a five-minute break at regular intervals throughout the day.

1   Sit in your chair with a straight spine. Place both feet flat on the floor, about hip-width apart. Place your right hand on your right knee and your left hand on your left knee. Your arms should be activated but not stiff.

2   Begin breathing in and out of your nose, filling your belly with each breath and releasing and pushing your navel to your spine. On the inhale, focus on filling your entire diaphragm. On the exhale, try pushing your breath to the back of your throat and down. (The exhale should sound like a hiss.) It's okay if you don't get the breath right the first couple of times; with practice, it will come. It is essential to create an internal awareness during yoga, not only to reap the greatest benefits but also to prevent injury to the body.

3   With each inhale, arch your spine forward, lifting your heart space upward and pulling your shoulders open and back. Keep your head still and shoulders relaxed. With each exhale, focus on pushing the breath out of your body while arching your spine back in the shape of a C. Roll your shoulders forward and tuck your navel toward your spine. Do this five times or as many times as you need to feel relaxed and tension-free.

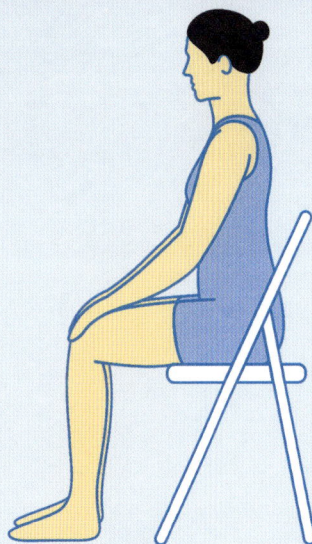

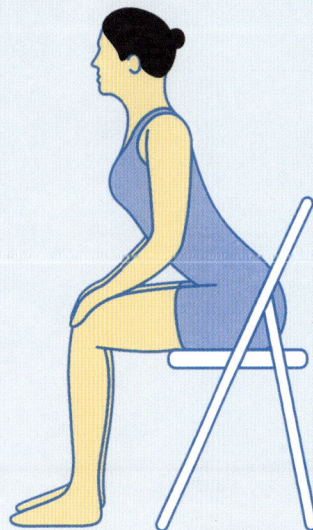

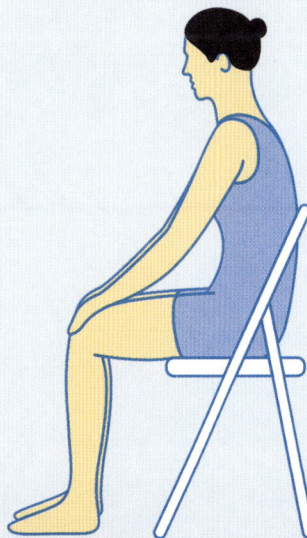

**Seated Spinal Twist (*Marichyasana III*)**

Twisting the spine has many benefits. It massages the abdominal muscles and organs, promoting digestion, and keeps the spine healthy. The spine builds up tension between the vertebrae that can cause stagnation and when we twist the spine we release the hidden tension.

1   Sit on the floor with your left leg outstretched and your right leg bent at the knee with your right foot on the floor. You can lift your butt cheeks and push them to the side so you really feel your sit bones—this helps to lengthen the spine.

2   Inhale, raising your arms up to lengthen your spine and twisting to the right toward the bent thigh, compressing your belly against the thigh. Allow your right hand to rest behind you as if it's a support for keeping your spine straight—you don't want to hunch over. Press your left elbow into the right thigh to increase the stretch.

3   If you feel comfortable, turn your neck toward the back of your right shoulder and allow your gaze to follow. Hold for five breaths. Repeat on the other side.

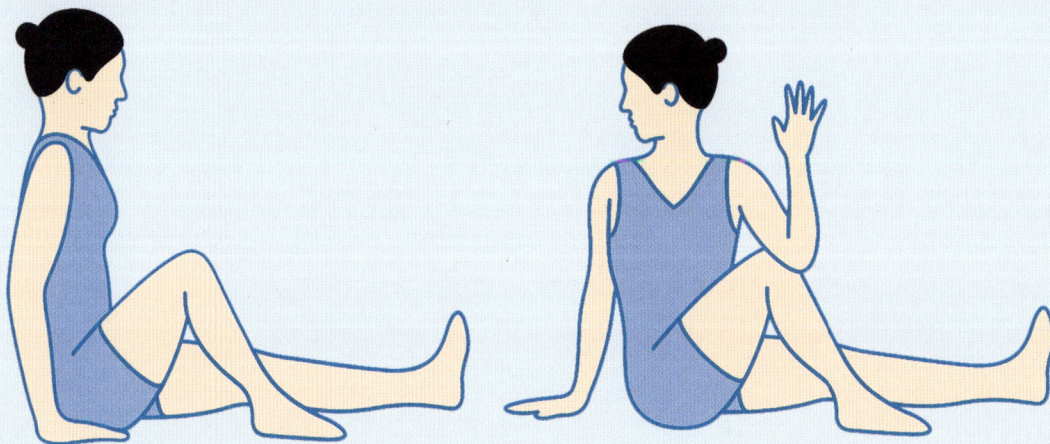

## Seated Forward Fold (*Paschimottanasana*)

Back pain and intense lower back tightness are pretty common afflictions. One of the easiest methods of relief is a Seated Forward Fold.

1  Sit on the floor with your legs stretched out in front of you. Make sure you can feel your sit bones under you and that you are balanced and sitting up tall.

2  Inhale, raising your arms up toward the sky and extending them as far as you can.

3  On the exhale, lift from your chest and fold forward from your hips toward your toes. Keep your chest lifted to protect your spine; don't collapse. If you can't reach your toes, that's okay, touch wherever you can: ankles, knees, thighs. If this is uncomfortable and your hamstrings are too tight, you can practice this pose using a blanket or yoga block under your tailbone. Hold the pose for five breaths and repeat as needed.

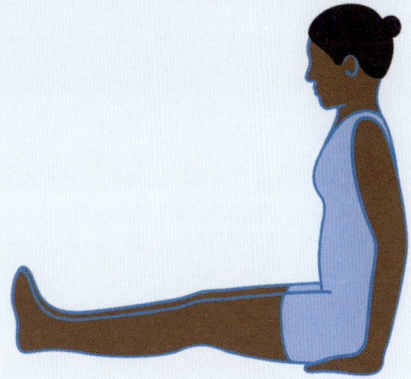

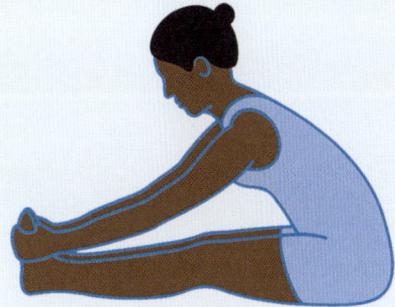

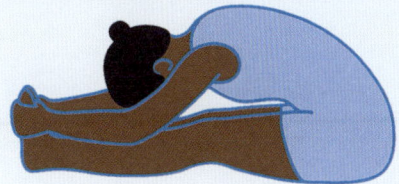

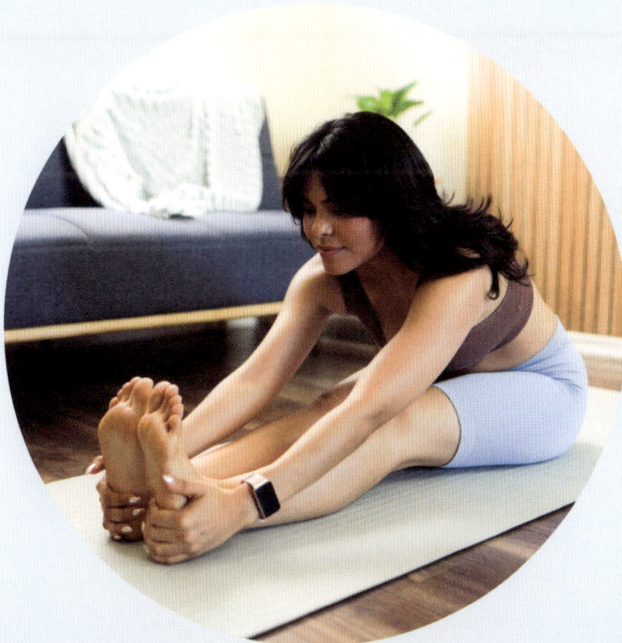

# Yoga poses to suit your needs

Certain yoga poses can be more beneficial for some individuals based on their unique physical and mental attributes, limitations, and goals. While yoga offers a wide range of benefits for both body and mind, tailoring a practice to individual needs ensures optimal results and minimizes the risk of injury.

## Slow-moving yoga poses

If you're prone to anxiety, over-exhaustion, and fatigue, or if you're a person who is highly energetic and erratic in nature, you will likely benefit most from exercises designed to ground you. Slow down your movement and take long pauses and breaks to offset what you are doing. Your body will love and thrive with extended practice of the Corpse Pose (see opposite)—give it a go for around 20 minutes.

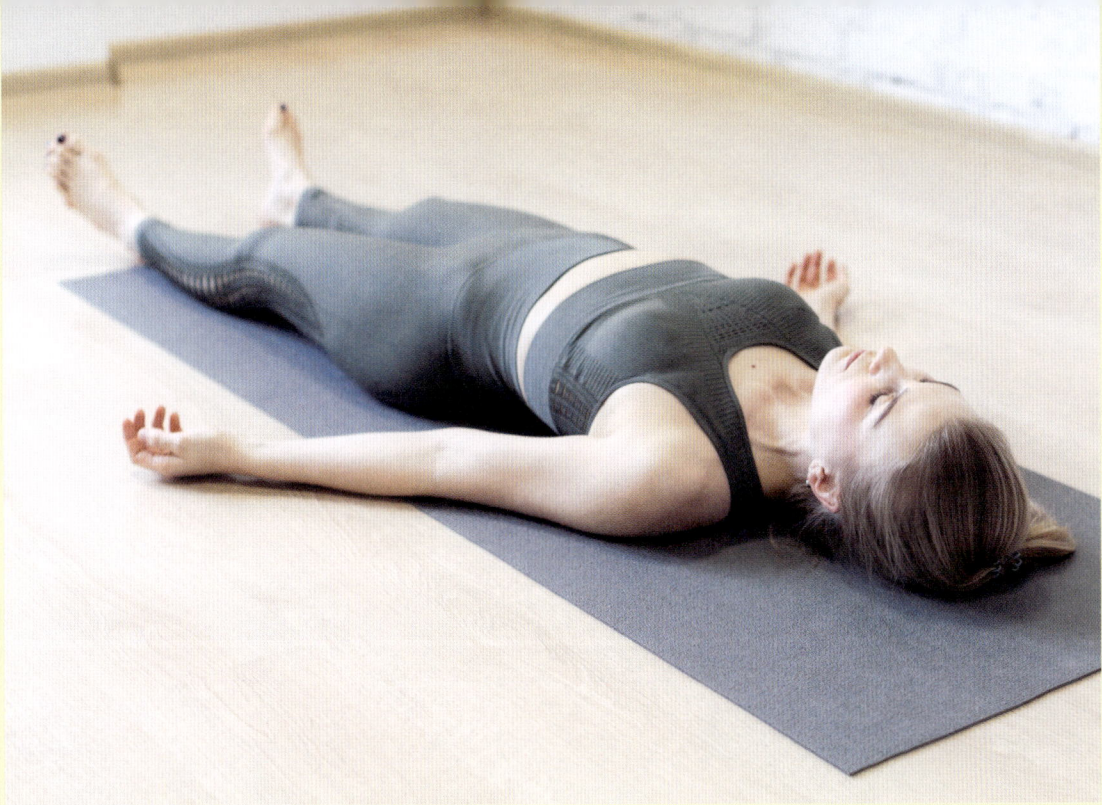

### Corpse Pose (*Savasana*)

**Benefits:** Repairs tissues and rejuvenates cells, relaxes muscles, improves breathing, and helps enhance meditation for those with an active mind.

1   Lie flat on the floor with your back connected to the ground and your arms relaxed by your sides, palms facing up. Your legs can be more than hip-width apart. Let your legs and feet roll out, letting go of any tension. This pose is about relaxation and slowing down.

2   Focus on your breath and let your thoughts come and go, sending breath and a healing light to each thought.

3   Slowly relax every muscle and nerve of your body, relaxing and releasing into the floor. Stay here and just breathe.

4   To come out of the pose, slowly wiggle your fingers and toes and wake up each part of your body before you decide to roll over and sit up.

**Mountain Pose (*Tadasana*)**

**Benefits:** Reduces anxiety and stress while grounding you to your root.

1  Stand with your arms at your sides. Roll your shoulders down your spine, releasing any tension in your head, neck, or shoulders. Distribute your weight evenly across both feet. Imagine being anchored and grounded by a string that starts at the top of your head and extends through your body, running equally down through both your inner ankles, outer ankles, big toes, and little toes.

2  Breathe in through your nose and out through your nose. Stay in Mountain Pose for two minutes.

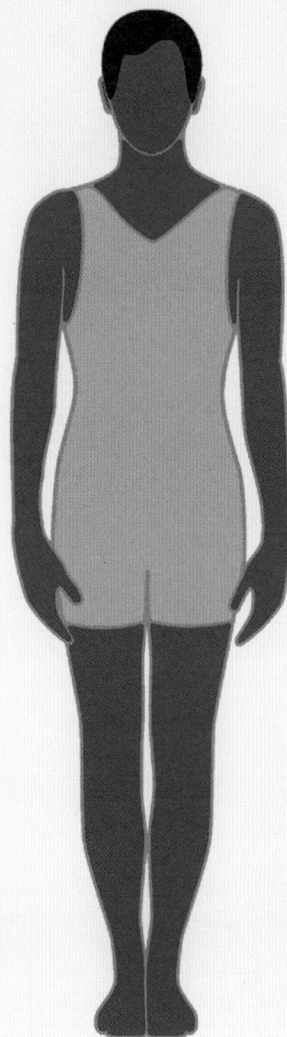

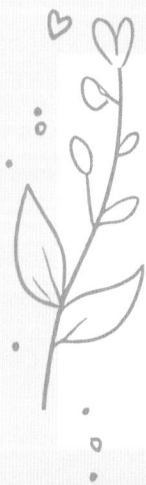

## ADDITIONAL ADVICE

People who regularly suffer from anxiety and emotional stress are also prone to constipation. To remedy this, poses and movements that include compression of the pelvis are very healing. Simple movements to help encourage the downward flow of energy are Forward Fold (see page 57), which can be done standing or sitting, and Seated Spinal Twist (see page 56).

## Tree Pose (*Vrksasana*)

**Benefits:** Helps to build strength while grounding and rooting you to the earth.

1   Stand in Mountain Pose (see opposite). Shift your weight onto your left foot and begin to bend your right knee, lifting your right foot off the floor. Using your core to keep your balance, reach down and clasp your right inner ankle. Draw your right foot alongside your left inner thigh. If this is too advanced, rest your right foot on the inside of your left calf or just below the knee—do not rest your foot directly on the knee.

2   Once you have gained your balance, shift your position so the center of your pelvis is directly over your left foot. Adjust your hips so your right hip and left hip are aligned. Rest your hands on your hips or, if you prefer, you can place them in front of your heart, palms pressing against each other in prayer position.

3   Once you are comfortable, extend your arms above your head with palms and fingers facing each other and then press them together in prayer position. To help you keep your balance, fix your gaze on an unmoving object or spot; this will help you to remain centered and keep the energy connected to the earth. Hold this pose for as long as possible or up to five minutes.

4   To come out of the pose, guide your ankle and foot back into Mountain Pose. Repeat on the other side.

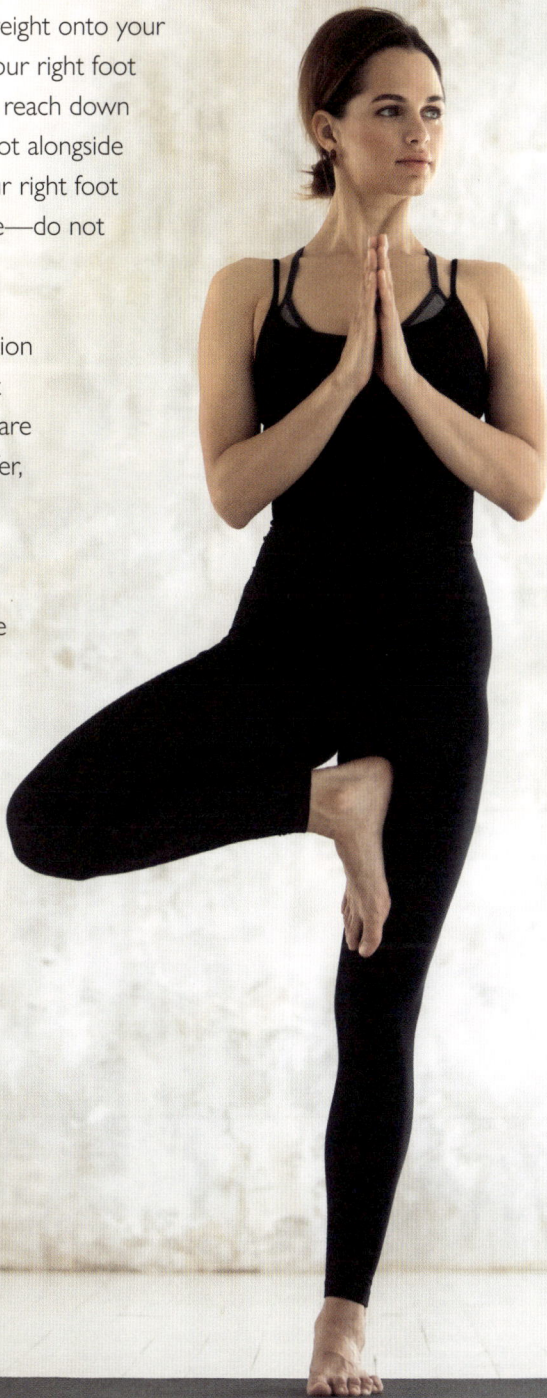

# Calming yoga poses

If you are a person who regularly gets fired up—whether you're a workaholic, overly ambitious, or simply have a quick temper—you will benefit the most from a calm, relaxing, and non-competitive movement routine. You may find it difficult to resist the urge to compete with others in your class or at the gym, but be as gentle as possible with yourself. It's also best to avoid hot yoga, hot Pilates, boxing, running in hot weather, and any other type of movement that could cause profuse sweating. Focus on activities that are calming and cooling to the body, such as taking walks barefoot through the grass in cool weather, swimming, surfing, snowboarding, and gentle yoga and use heart- and hip-opening poses to release any trapped heat in the body.

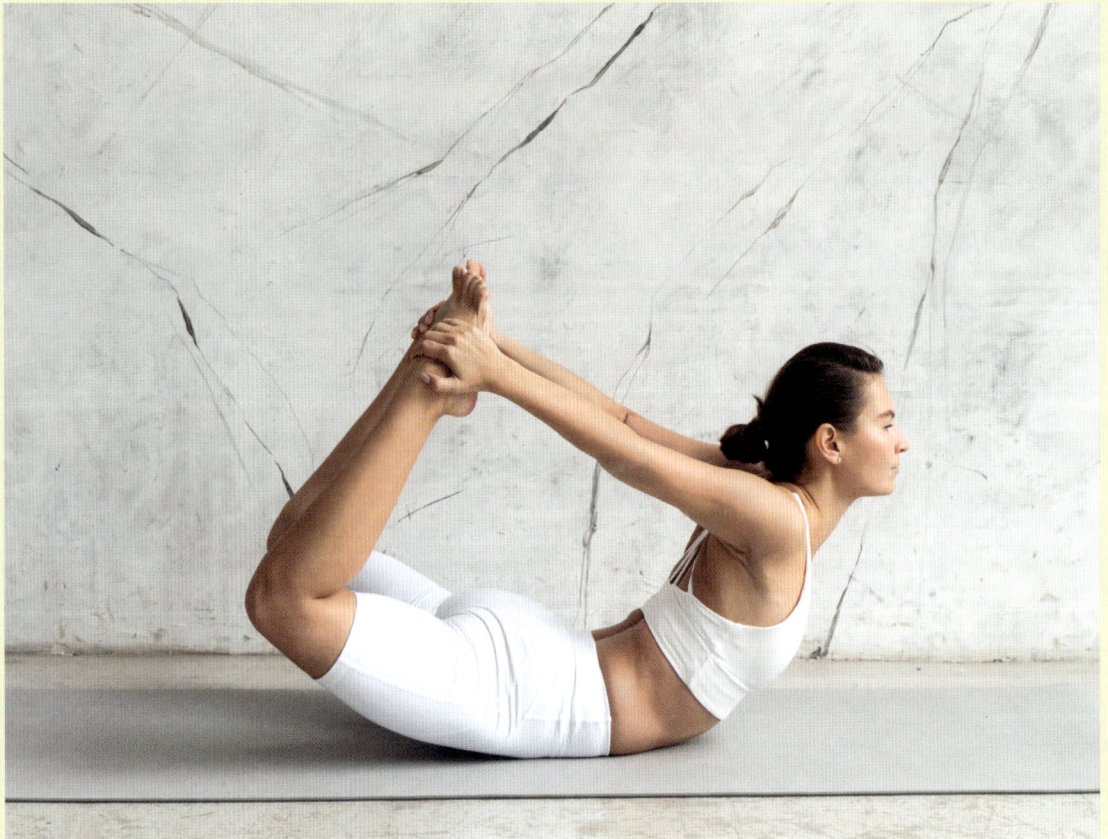

**Bow Pose (*Dhanurasana*)**

**Benefits:** Helps to open up the heart center, releasing any
stagnant or trapped heat.

1    Lie face-down on the floor with your arms relaxed by your sides,
     palms facing up. Bend your knees and exhale, bringing your heels
     toward your butt. Focus on sending the heels as close to your butt as possible.
     Make sure that your knees are hip-width apart (the distance will vary from person
     to person). Reach back with both hands and clasp your ankles, making sure you are
     holding onto your ankles and not your feet.

2    On the inhale, strongly push the energy from your torso up and back, lifting your
     heels away from your butt and your thighs away from the floor. Your head, neck,
     torso, and shoulders should be off the floor. You should feel the back bend at this
     point. Don't tighten your back muscles.

3    Softly send the inhale and exhale into your chest, releasing any tension and
     gently rolling your shoulders down and back to open your heart even more.
     Breathe into your back, as breathing may be slightly difficult with the pressure
     of your body on your belly. Don't hold your breath; the breath helps you open
     and stretch into tight areas of the body to release pain and heat. Try to stay
     in this pose for 20 seconds.

4    To come out of the pose, release on the exhale and relax your body, head turned
     to the left, hands folded under your face. Lie quietly for a minute. Repeat two
     more times.

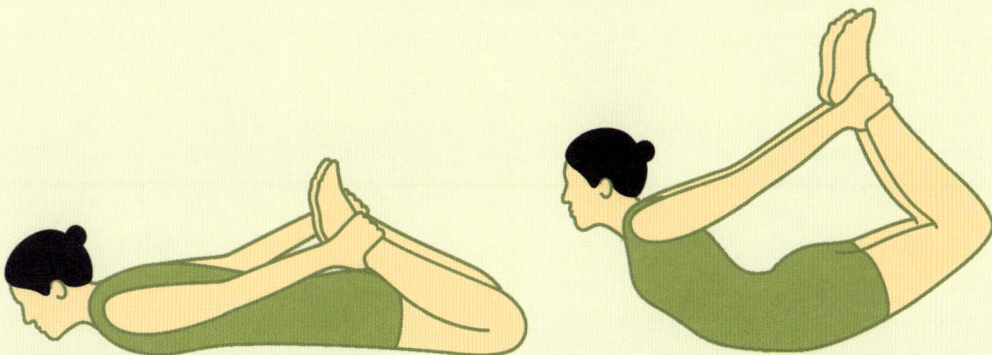

### Fish Pose (*Matsyasana*)

**Benefits**: Strengthens the upper back muscles and stretches the front of the body and hip flexors.

1   Lie flat on your back with both legs extended straight in front of your body and your arms relaxed.

2   Press both forearms and elbows into the floor, lifting your chest upward to the sky and creating a slight arch in your upper back. The goal is to create an arch in your upper back in order to release tension in the chest.

3   Tilt your head back toward the floor and place the crown of your head on the floor. (If your head does not reach the floor or you need more support, use a yoga block, bolster, or blanket to support the back of your head.) This will draw the energy of your shoulder blades down and back and lift your upper torso off the floor. Use your forearms and hands to stabilize your body and keep the pressure off your head. Press upward through your heels to keep your thighs engaged and active.

4   Inhale and exhale for ten breaths, holding for five at the top of each breath.

5   To come out of the pose, press firmly into your forearms, allowing your head to release off the floor. Exhale, bring your torso to the floor and draw your knees up and in toward your chest. Wrap your arms around your knees and give them a hug. Relax and repeat two more times.

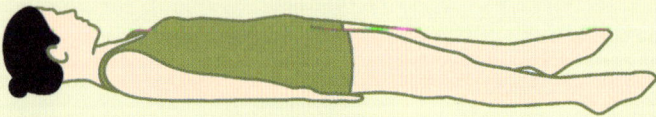

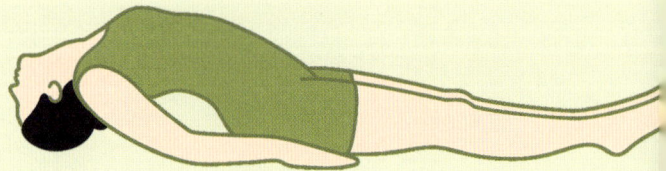

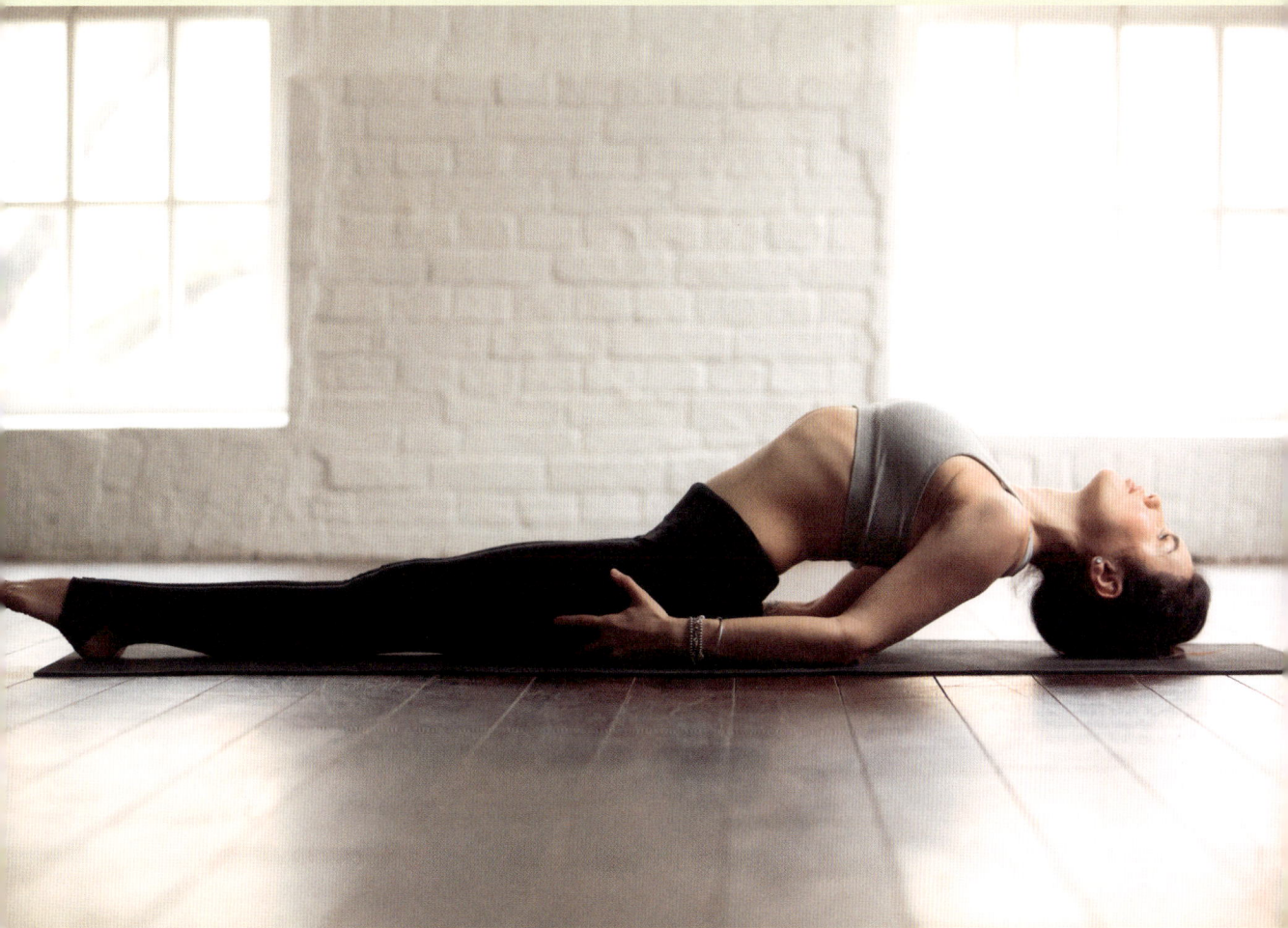

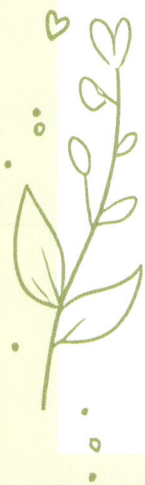

## ADDITIONAL ADVICE

People with a high energy level benefit greatly from meditation and earthing. Earthing is the practice of connecting with the earth by walking barefoot across it, which helps to cool and calm the body. Try to do a walking meditation around your yard, block, or somewhere outside your home for at least ten minutes once a day at sundown. You don't only have to walk across grass to feel the earth, walking on pavement or cement might feel weird at first but this is an effective form of earthing as well. Focus on your breathing, release your thoughts, and connect your body to the earth.

## Invigorating yoga poses

If you're a person who lives a sedentary, grounded life, you will likely benefit the most from yoga that is invigorating, warm, and fast-paced. A lack of high-energy movement can lead to severe lethargy, weight gain, and depression, but yoga combats this by invigorating a person's energy and releasing endorphins that combat mood swings and depression. Kickboxing, high-intensity interval training (HIIT), hot Pilates, and warm infrared yoga are also optimal for someone like this. If you tend to be sluggish in the morning, try to get your movement in between the hours of 6 a.m. and 10 a.m., as this will help sustain an energized state and keep you motivated throughout the day.

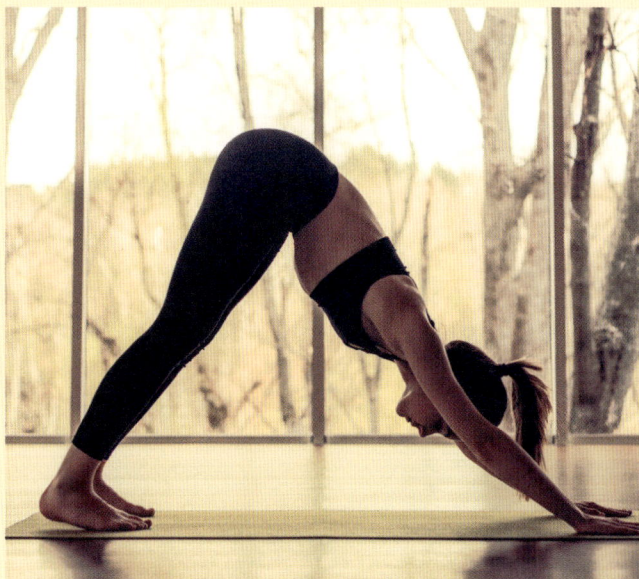

## ADDITIONAL ADVICE

If yoga is not your favorite form of exercise, find a physical hobby that you love and do it daily. Biking, dancing, and running are great alternatives. If you find yourself wanting to be more sedentary for no apparent reason, this is a sign that you need to up your daily movement.

## Downward-facing Dog (*Adho Mukha Svanasana*)

**Benefits:** Helps to energize the entire body and rev up cardiovascular energy, which will get the heat moving throughout the body.

1   Kneel on a yoga mat with your knees hip-width apart, your arms straight, and your palms on the floor. Spread your palms wide and stack your shoulders over your wrists. This is Tabletop Pose. You will need to keep your knees hip-width apart throughout the entire pose.

2   When you're comfortable, curl your toes under and lift your knees off the ground. Raise your body up, lifting from your pelvis, and straighten your legs. Press down to send the energy out of your heels and try to place both heels on the yoga mat. You may need to readjust your arms and walk the palms of your hands out in front of your shoulders slightly.

3   Imagine a string pulling your belly toward your back, breathe deeply, and hold the inverted V position. Stay in this pose for 20 breaths.

4   To come out of the pose, bend your knees and fold back into Tabletop Pose.

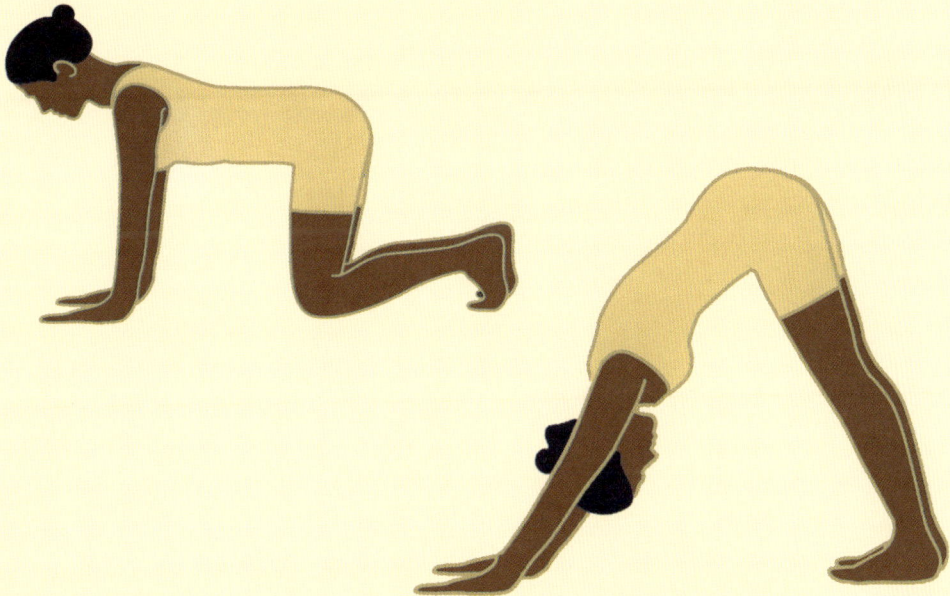

### Downward-facing Dog (*Adho Mukha Svanasana*)
### to Plank Position (*Kumbhakasana*)

**Benefits:** Builds core and upper body strength (but if you struggle with Plank Position, holding Downward-facing Dog for an extended period will also build your core and upper body strength).

1   Starting from Downward-facing Dog (see page 67), inhale and draw your torso forward until your arms are perpendicular (at right angles) to the floor and your shoulders are directly over your wrists. Your torso should be parallel to the floor, as if you were doing a push-up. Resist your butt going up toward the ceiling and lengthen your tailbone back toward your heels. Lift your head up and look straight down at the floor, keeping the back of your neck relaxed and your throat soft.

2   Once you are comfortable in Plank Position, roll back and forth from Plank to Downward-facing Dog, increasing your pace and bringing up your heart rate. Do this for two minutes straight, no break.

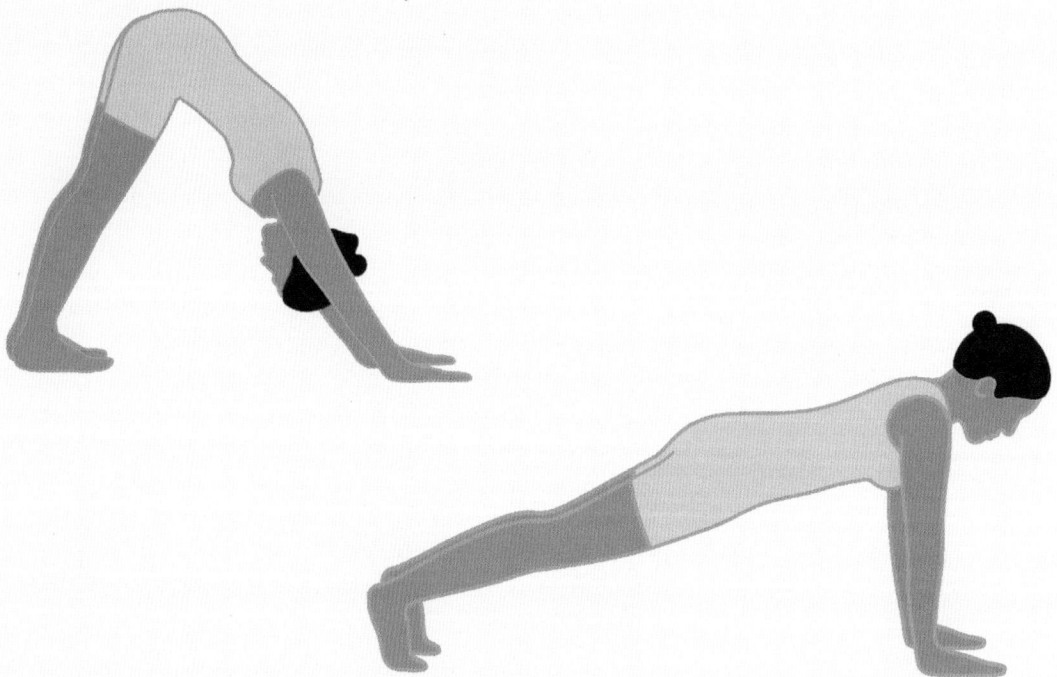

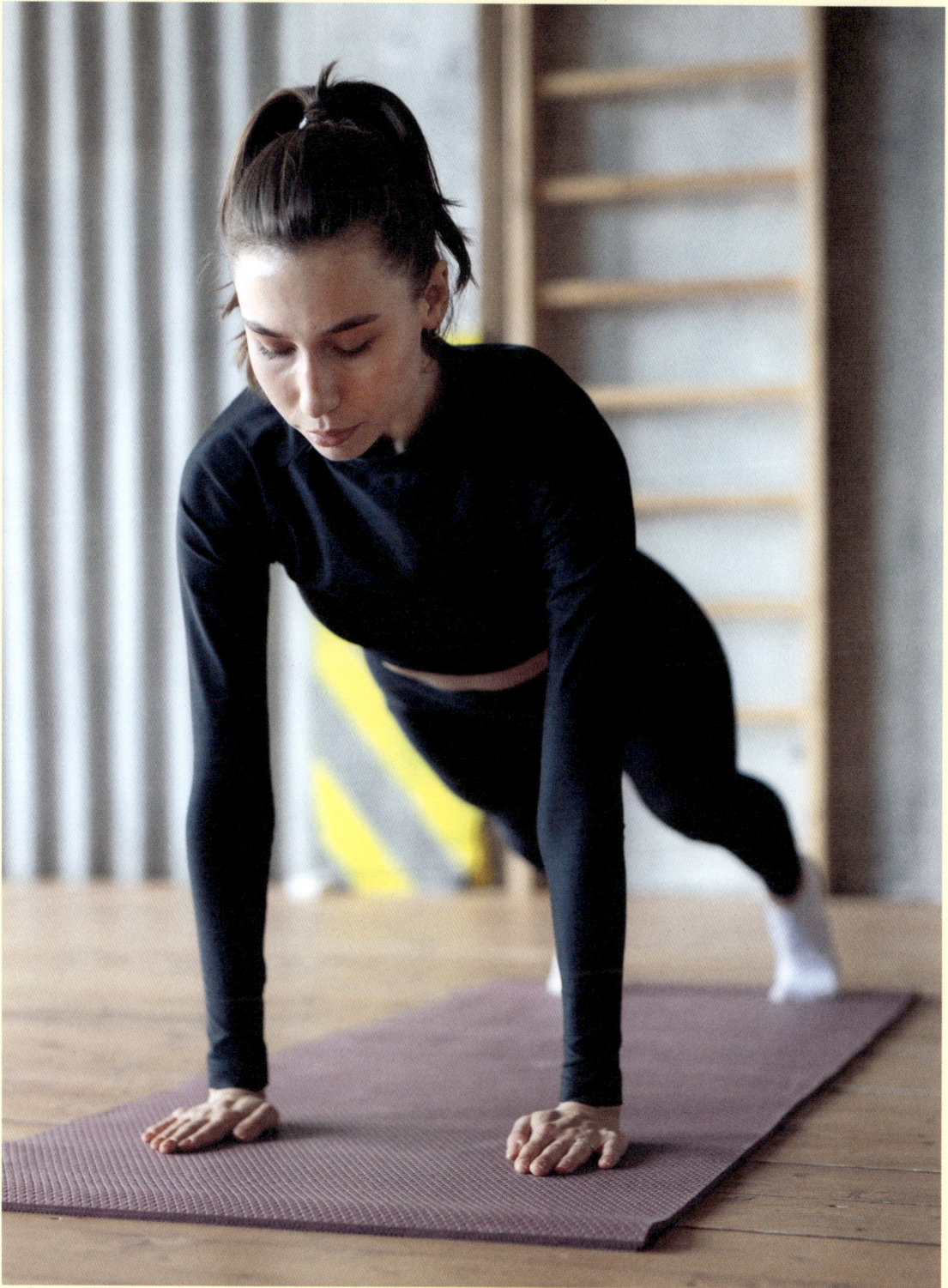

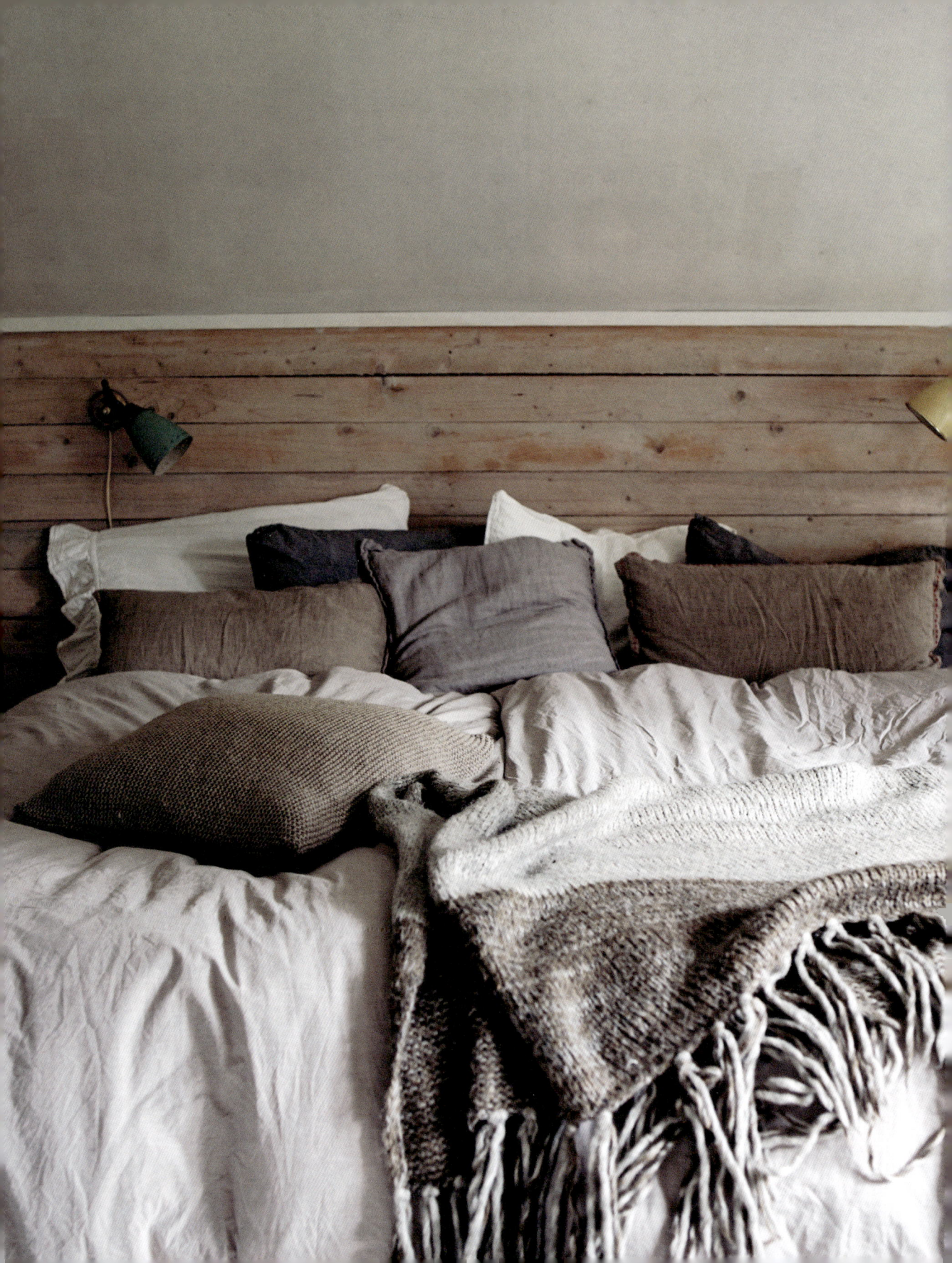

# Chapter 3

# Rest and Recharge

Discover natural remedies that enable true relaxation and peace of mind, from adjusting your sleep environment to using CBD oil to create calm.

# The importance of rest

What many people don't realize is that sleep is one of the cornerstones of wellbeing, along with diet and exercise. We may be aware that regularly eating junk food and not exercising affects our physical and mental wellbeing, but we may not make the same connection with not getting enough sleep.

Everyone will at some point experience periods when they find it difficult to relax and rest. These are most often triggered by a stressful event, but it can also be caused by illness, whether physical or psychological. While some illnesses can cause insomnia, sleep and the physiological functions of the body are so intertwined that many medical conditions can also be exacerbated by, or be a result of, sleep deprivation. Although this is an emerging field in research, with new discoveries being made all the time, it is known that sleep is closely linked to all the body's physiological systems, and so when sleep is disrupted, it is inevitable that we don't function at our best, emotionally, mentally, and physically.

## Pairing mindfulness with relaxation

When we practice mindfulness, we focus our attention on the here and now, registering how we feel and recognizing actions and behaviors that are helpful for achieving true relaxation, as well as those that are unhelpful. Once we become aware of this, we usually find ourselves intentionally choosing to do more of the helpful and less of the unhelpful. Making some simple changes can create small shifts, each contributing to an overall improvement. However, everyone is different, so you should experiment and explore what you notice about your habits and behavior, and how they support or affect your sleep quality.

In general, eight hours of sleep is usually quoted for adults; children and young adults will need more and the elderly less. However, it is important not to get too hooked on numbers, particularly if you do have trouble sleeping, since there may be a tendency to constantly measure how you are doing and then feel disappointed if you are falling short. This may create additional anxiety about sleeping, and that is unhelpful. Mindfulness helps us to let go of particular expectations and of striving toward a particular goal, and instead helps us to be okay with the way things actually are.

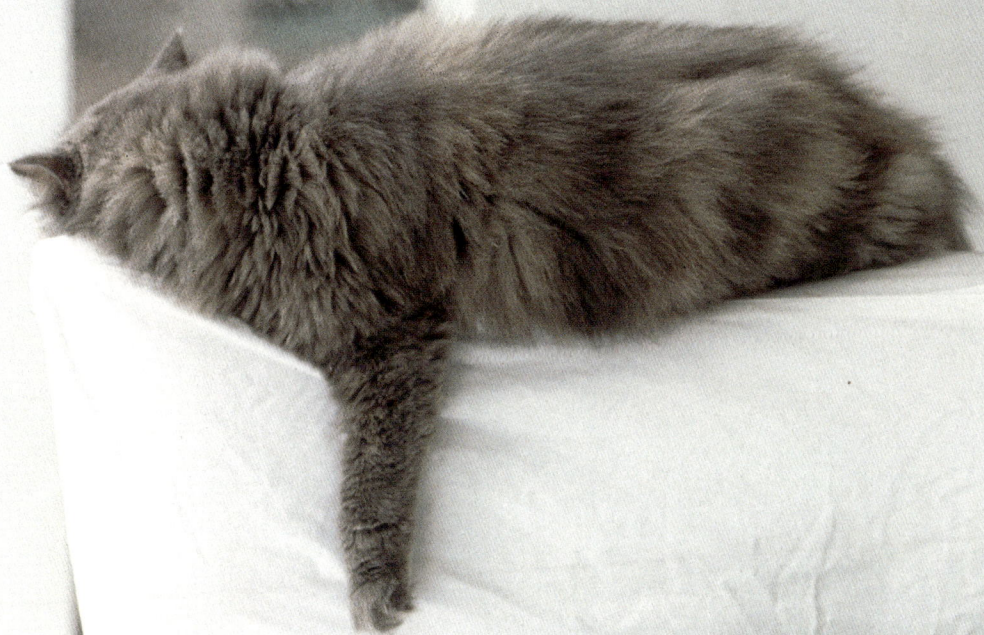

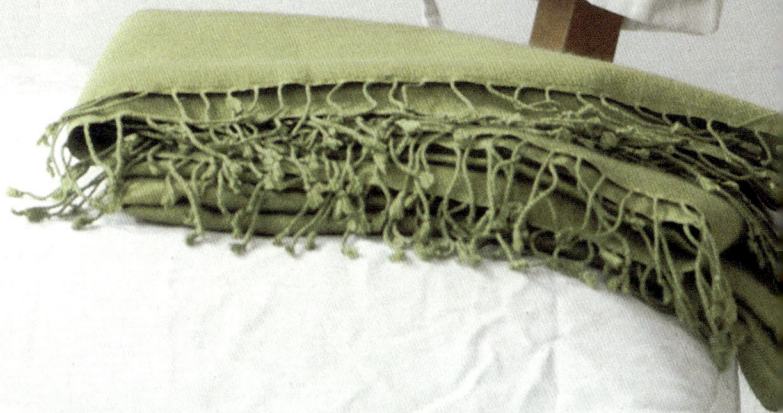

# How sleep benefits us

It's often said that diet, exercise, and sleep are the three foundational pillars to good health and wellbeing. While many of us understand the importance of eating a healthy, balanced diet and of keeping fit, we are perhaps less familiar with how important sleep is.

We've all experienced the effects of too little sleep: what it means for our mood, focus, and concentration, and also how it affects us physically—we have less energy, and feel tired and groggy. However, the importance of sleep and the consequences of being sleep-deprived go beyond this.

Sleep influences all the major systems in our body, and those systems in turn influence our sleep. Insufficient sleep can disrupt bodily functions that affect how we

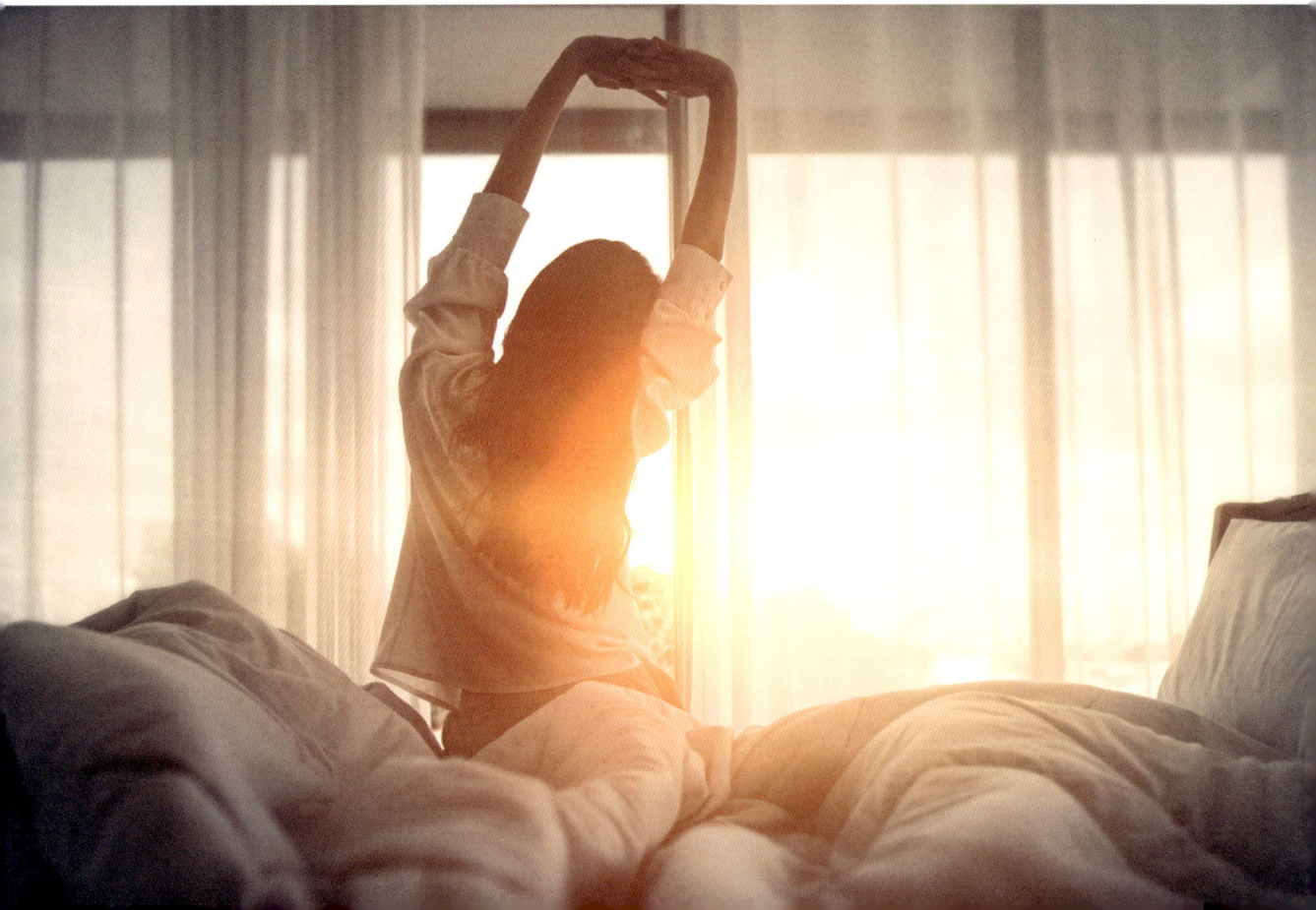

think and behave, and how we think and behave can disrupt our sleep. Therefore problems with sleeping can quickly become a vicious cycle.

At its simplest, sleep plays an important role in:

- Creating a healthy immune system
- Repairing muscle
- Consolidating learning and memory
- Regulating growth and appetite through the release of certain hormones
- Regulating mood and emotion

Sufficient sleep is essential to our wellbeing, both physically and emotionally, so it is not surprising that when we are deprived of it, we feel the impact in all areas of our life. There is plenty of evidence that poor-quality or too little sleep can have serious consequences for our physical and mental health.

## The science behind it

Whether we are awake or asleep depends on activity in specific areas of the brain. The part of the brain that promotes wakefulness also inhibits the part that promotes sleep activity, and vice versa. The shift between the different areas is caused by internal factors such as the circadian rhythm and the release of hormones, and is usually self-regulating. The drive to sleep increases the longer we are awake, and as we sleep it abates so that it is near zero when we wake.

Sleep, or more officially the Sleep Cycle, is made up of different stages of REM (rapid eye movement) and n-REM (non-rapid eye movement) sleep. Each cycle lasts about 90 minutes and is repeated three to six times each night. However, this cycle may be disrupted by stimulants such as coffee, nicotine, and alcohol, as well as by medical conditions and sleep deprivation. Find out more about the stages of the Sleep Cycle on pages 76–77.

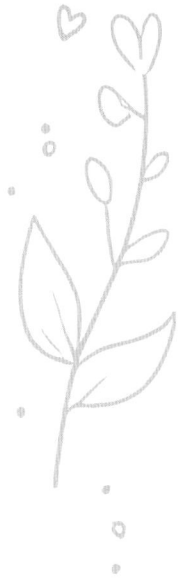

# THE SLEEP CYCLE

We usually spend about 75 percent of the night in n-REM and 25 percent in REM sleep. Each of the different stages is as important as the others, and it is believed that the right balance of all the stages is crucial for restful and restorative sleep, which promotes learning, memory, and growth processes such as cell formation and repair, and regulates mood and the ability to concentrate.

## N-REM

Characterized by a reduction in physiological activity in the body, sleep gradually becomes deeper and the brain waves slow, along with the breath, heart rate, and blood pressure. Although the following are listed as separate stages, they actually merge into one another.

- N1 (Stage 1): Typically lasts one to seven minutes, when we are hovering between being awake and falling asleep. If we are asleep, it is very light. We may experience sudden muscle jerks preceded by a falling sensation.
- N2 (Stage 2): Lasts about 10–25 minutes and signifies the onset of sleep. Eye movement stops, breath and heart rate become more regular, and body temperature drops. We have disengaged from our surroundings. Brain waves become slower, with occasional bursts of rapid activity. Spontaneous periods of muscle tension are interspersed with periods of muscle relaxation.
- N3 (Stage 3): Typically lasts 20–40 minutes and is also called Slow Wave Sleep (SWS). This is our deepest and most restorative sleep, and is believed to be associated with bodily recovery, certain types of learning, and changes to the central nervous system. Children experience the greatest amount of N3 sleep, which decreases with age. The longer someone has been awake, the more N3 sleep they get once N3 sleep occurs.

It is harder to wake someone in N3 (Stage 3) sleep than in any other, since the brain is less responsive to external stimuli. If we are awakened in this stage, we may feel groggy and disoriented for a while.

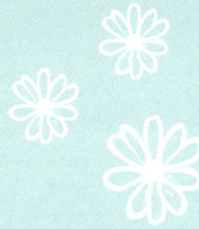

## REM

REM sleep usually occurs about 90 minutes after falling asleep. It recurs every 90 minutes or so, and lasts longer as the night progresses. There is intense brain activity similar to when we are awake. This is when we are most likely to dream.

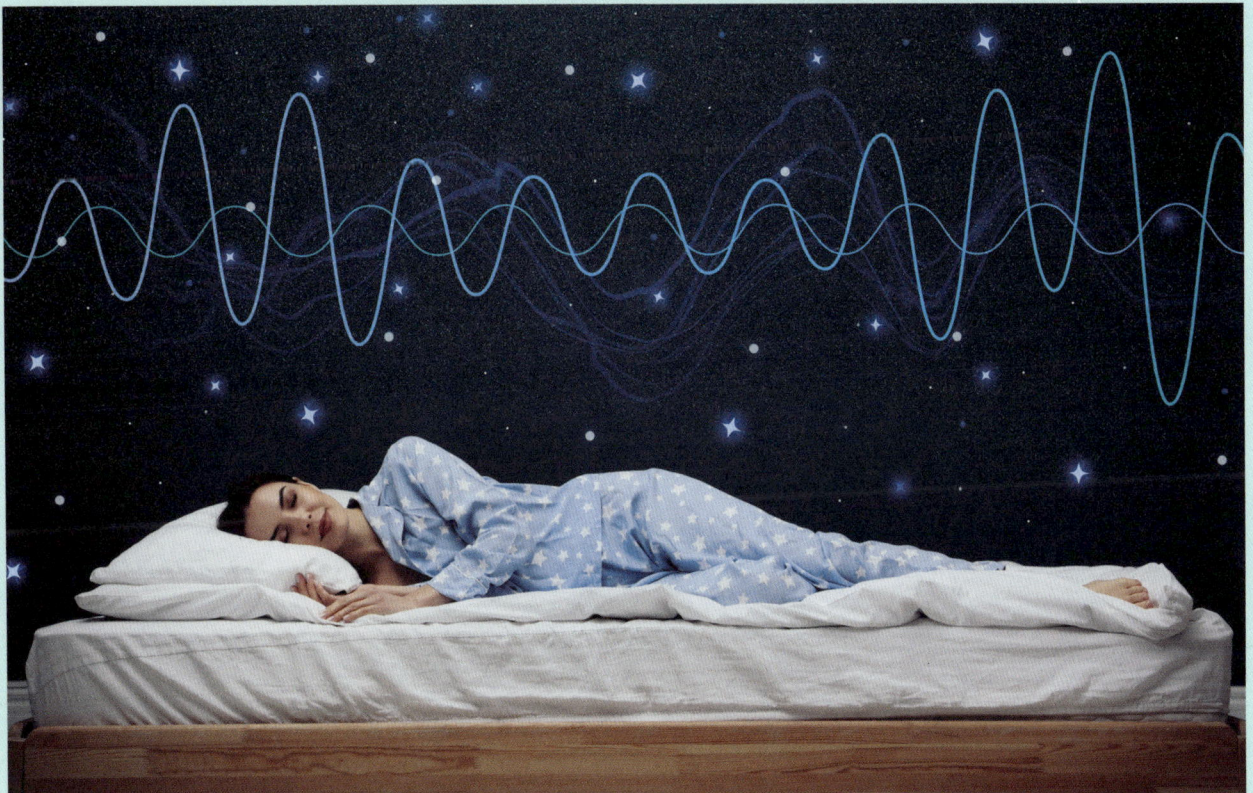

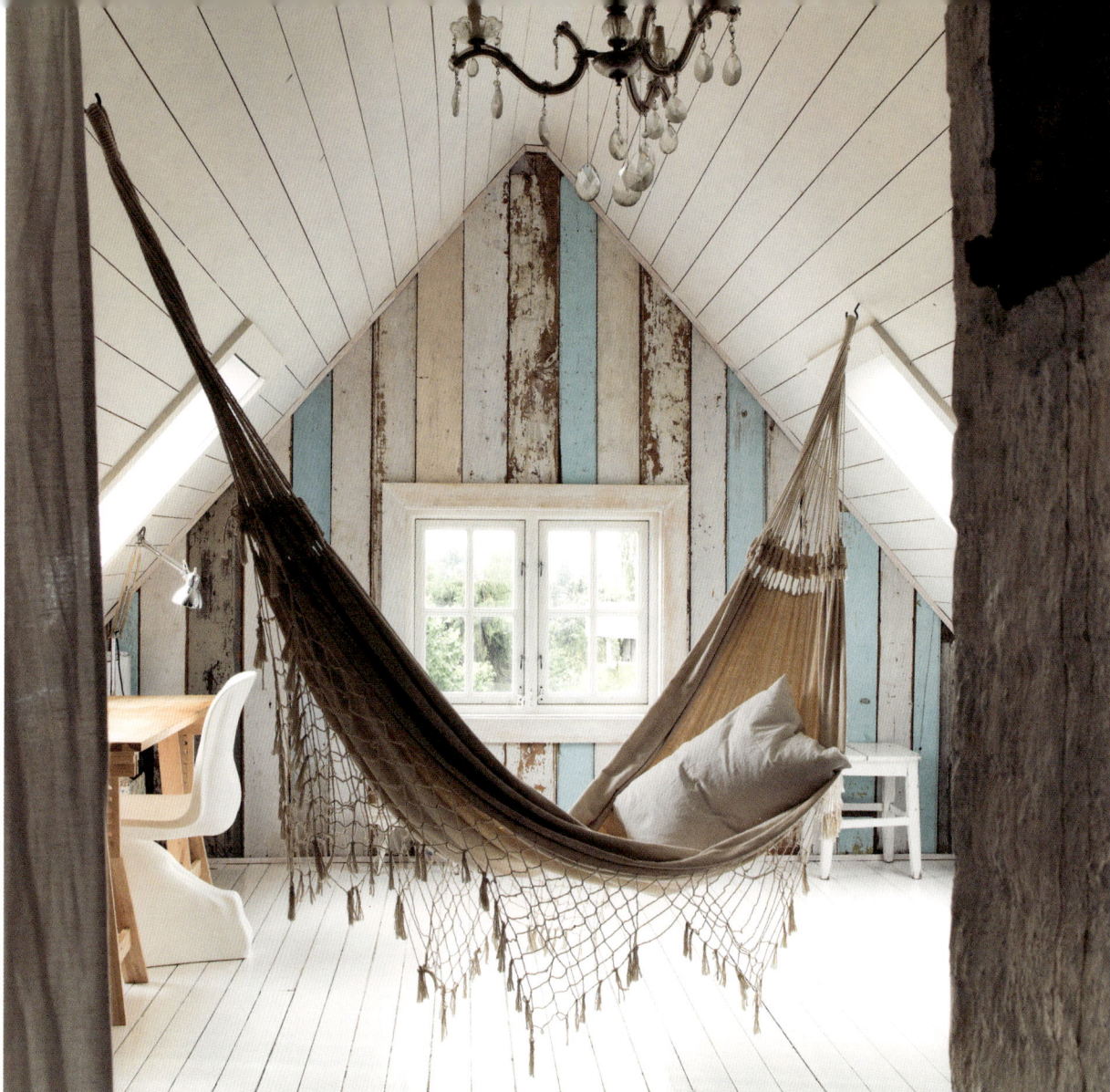

# What stops us from resting

Many factors affect our ability to sleep. Some are beyond our control, and it becomes a question of learning how to live with their consequences, but others are related to lifestyle, so we can do something about them.

## Age

As we get older, our total sleep time and the period we spend in deep Slow Wave Sleep (see page 76) decreases. Since we are less likely to be woken by external stimuli when we are in deep sleep, the number of times we wake up increases and sleep becomes fragmented. Once we are awake it also takes us longer to fall back to sleep. This may all be caused by lifestyle changes, such as retirement, as well as increased health problems and the side-effects of medication, but many people find that they need less sleep as they become older, too. Women may experience night sweats and poorer sleep overall with the onset of the menopause.

## Medical disorders

Those that affect sleep include apnea (when a person's airway becomes blocked or obstructed, resulting in shallow breathing or even a temporary stop in breathing, which disrupts sleep), mental-health disorders such as depression and anxiety, obesity, and pain.

## Work

Shift work can be particularly disruptive, but working long or irregular hours can adversely affect the body's natural rhythms.

## Environment

This might be a room that is too warm, external noise (airplanes, neighbors, traffic), or perhaps a snoring partner or one who also has difficulty sleeping.

## Travel

Crossing time zones disrupts our internal body clock, which regulates sleep and waking.

## Stress

This could be caused by relationship problems, work (or lack of work after retirement), bereavement, and young children, among other factors. Worrying can keep us awake and stress degrades melatonin, which is essential for sleep.

## Insomnia

This condition is when you have trouble falling asleep or staying asleep, when you wake very early, and/or when you don't feel satisfied with the quality of your sleep. If this persists for a month or more, it becomes a chronic condition. People experiencing insomnia often feel that their mind is racing, and get caught up in spirals of worry and negative thinking. This state of arousal keeps them awake.

## Lifestyle

Partying late, binge-watching your favorite show, or spending long hours at a computer, plus drinking alcohol or caffeine or taking other stimulants are all factors that can affect sleep. Plus, when we have trouble sleeping, we may inadvertently employ strategies that make it worse, thereby fueling rather than reducing our sleep debt.

# Strategies for better sleep

Although we can feel powerless in the face of poor sleep, there are some simple changes we can make to ensure that we are supporting rather than undermining our body's internal sleep systems.

People commonly report that implementing good sleeping habits is helpful. However, if you find your sleep does not improve despite making and maintaining lifestyle changes, it is recommended that you consult your physician.

## Cool down

Body temperature plays an important role in sleep. We fall asleep as our body temperature drops, and a lower body temperature also helps us to stay asleep before it begins to rise in the early hours as we awaken. You can encourage a drop in body temperature deliberately by taking a hot bath or shower about an hour before bedtime and then making sure your environment is cool (about 63°F/17°C). As the body cools, you will begin to feel sleepy. Ideally, exercise no less than four hours before going to bed, to avoid elevating your core temperature.

## Environment

Sleep in a cool, dark room that is free of technology and has a comfortable bed. Turn any clocks to the wall to avoid watching the minutes in the early hours.

## Don't spend too long in bed

If our mood is low, we may retreat to bed rather than face the world. However, going to bed too early means repeated awakenings and a much shallower sleep, and we thereby miss out on restorative Slow Wave Sleep (see page 76).

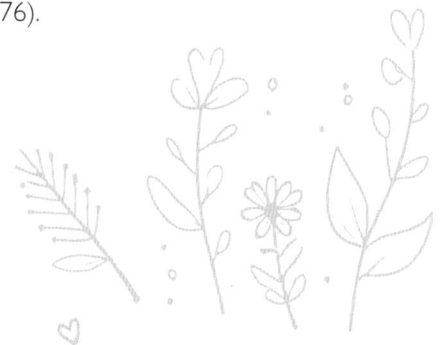

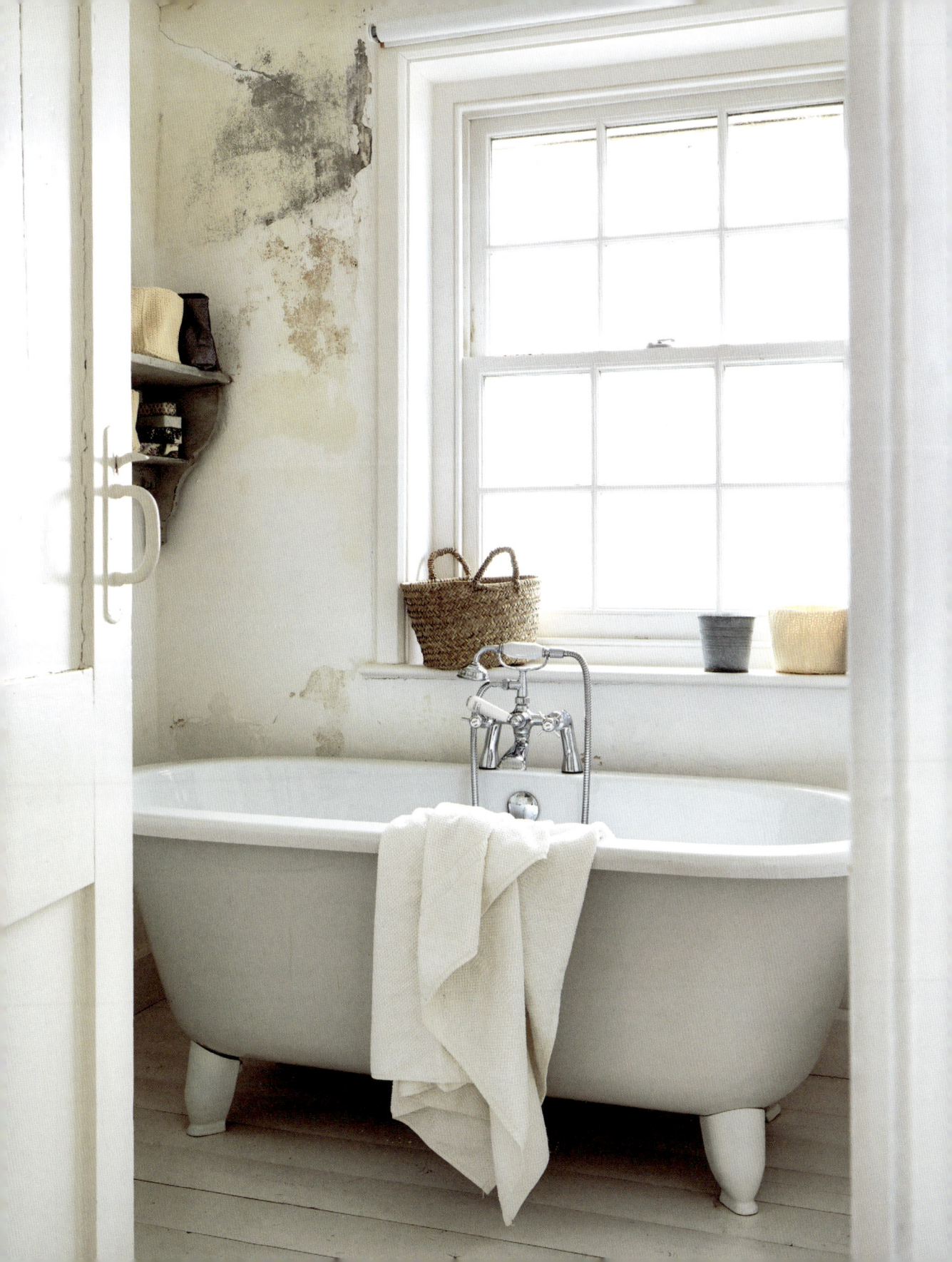

## Keep to a regular schedule

Stabilize your circadian rhythm by going to bed and getting up at the same time, even at weekends and when on vacation.

## Go to bed when you are sleepy

Listen to your body, and go to bed when you are sleepy. Likewise, don't go to bed before you are sleepy.

## Avoid stimulants

Alcohol, caffeine, nicotine, and other stimulants are best avoided in the evening and perhaps even in the afternoon. Notice how you are affected. It is important to check ingredients—you may be surprised how prevalent caffeine is. It can be found in chocolate, many sodas, and even energy drinks.

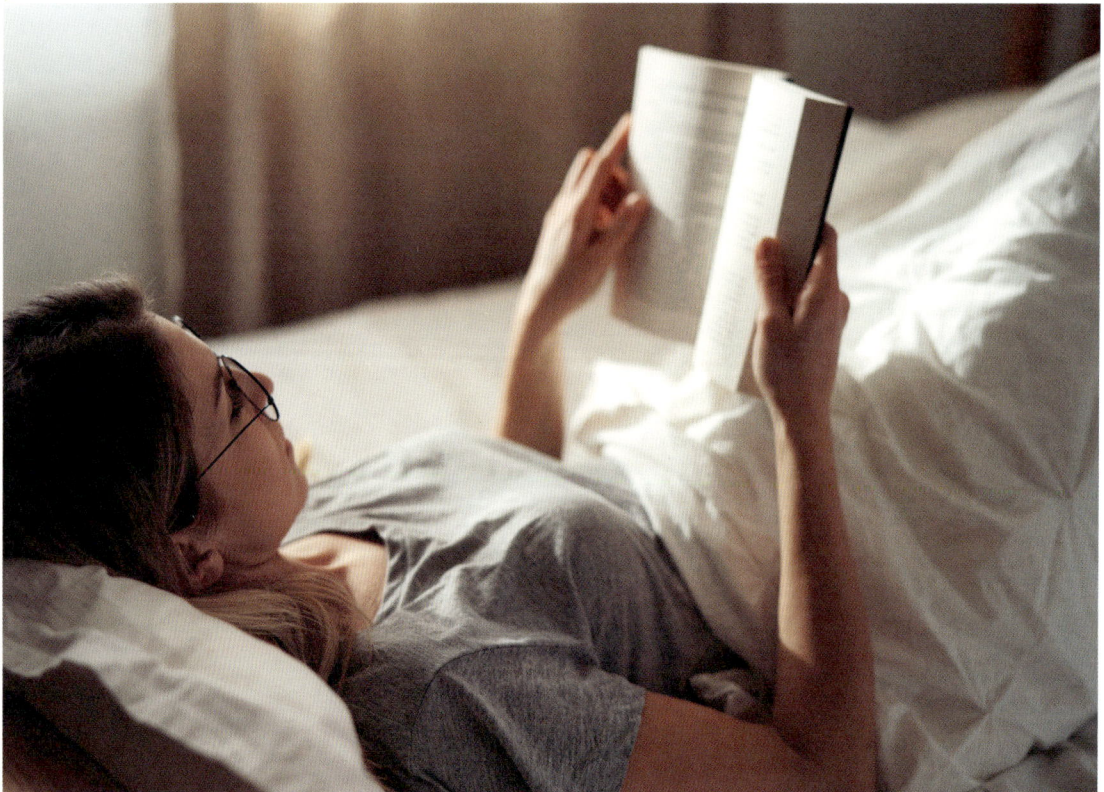

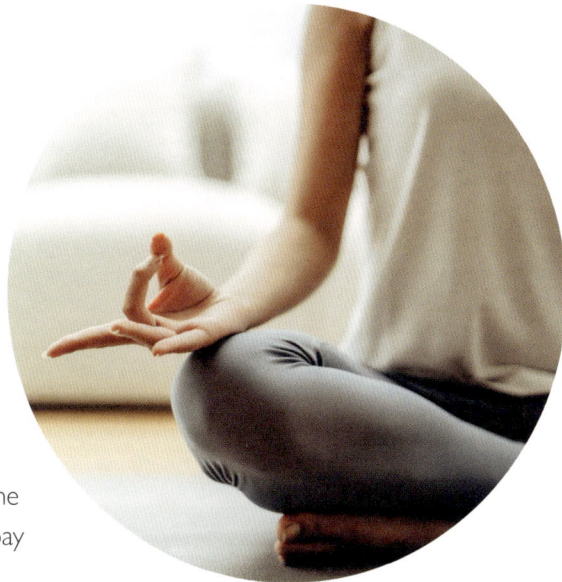

## Notice what you eat

Certain types of food eaten too near bedtime can affect your sleep, but they can affect everyone differently, so if you think food may be a factor pay attention to what you eat.

## Avoid trying to sleep

Actively trying to fall asleep will only make you more awake, particularly because you may begin to feel anxious that you are not falling asleep. If you are awake, be awake. Read, get up, meditate, or do some yoga or other calming activity.

## Reduce screen time

Avoid screen time (including television and cell phones) an hour before bedtime, if possible.

## Protect your wind-down time

Notice what helps you to move from the busy-ness of the day to winding down toward bedtime. Avoid or keep to a minimum activities that keep you buzzing. However, notice if there is a sense of striving when it comes to doing particular activities or behaving in a particular way, with the expectation that they will lead to a good night's sleep. This is unhelpful, too.

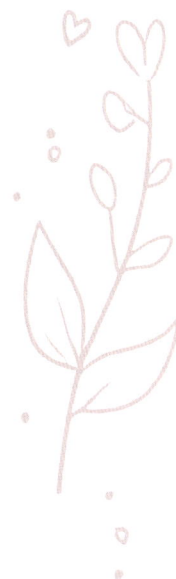

# Mindful attitudes to sleep

When we practice mindfulness, we consciously cultivate certain attitudes in the way we pay attention to our experience. These attitudes also arise from meditation practices and help us, ultimately, to achieve a peaceful, rest-enhancing state.

## Non-striving

We often have a goal in mind—we "should" be able to fall asleep instantly, or we "should" be able to stop worrying or sleep for eight hours. When we are striving for an outcome, we constantly measure and judge ourselves according to how well or badly we think we are doing. This is unhelpful, and sets us up for disappointment and frustration. It is counterproductive to try to force ourselves to sleep (it will only increase anxiety and tension); instead, we simply focus on our experience in the present moment.

## Letting go

Being willing to let go of wanting to fix or change our experience (often to make it better) and instead acknowledge how it is (even if we don't like it) is the first step in accepting things as they are. Being willing to let things unfold requires us to let go of wanting to control our experience. Falling asleep requires us to let go of effort and striving.

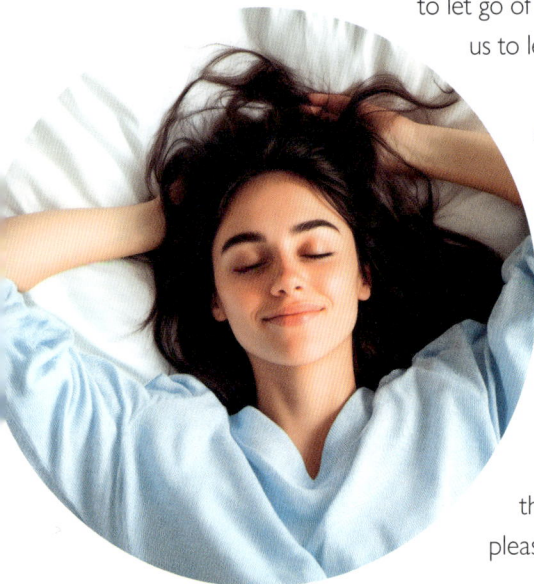

## Acceptance

This is an active state of acknowledging how things actually are rather than resisting them or pushing them away (our usual mode). Resisting the way things are takes a lot of energy, and usually involves blaming ourselves, others, or a particular situation. If we can drop the stories we are telling ourselves about "not sleeping" that are fueling our anxiety, we are left with simply being awake. If we are awake, it is better to accept that we are not sleepy, and get up and do something pleasurable or satisfying.

## Trust

This is tied very closely to non-striving, cultivating a willingness to give it a go as best you can for a reasonable period (several weeks is recommended). Change takes time and doesn't follow a straight trajectory of improvement. Some nights we might sleep worse than others, but that doesn't mean it will last forever. The body is primed to self-regulate, and if we can support those systems with good habits, the body will find its natural rhythm.

## Patience

We are working with patterns that we have built up over many years, and it takes time to learn to relate to things differently. It's not helpful to expect perfection—we must just do the best we can considering our circumstances. Change often comes about through making small alterations to our lives, each one influencing the next, and even sleeping an extra hour or not creating additional suffering by worrying about being awake can transform how we are feeling.

## Curiosity

When we are curious, we are interested and we want to find out more; to do that, we must pay attention and move in closer. It seems counterintuitive to move toward something that we don't like or that we see as a threat, but changing the way we perceive our experience is crucial. By consciously moving toward things, we learn to become less reactive and better able to respond to whatever is occurring. By becoming interested in our experience (thoughts, emotions, physical sensations, and behavior), we notice what is present and let go of the need to know why.

## Beginner's mind

Very often we have a fixed idea about the way something will be, and we see things through our own filters of memory and experience. This saps the vitality from everyday living, since we are not open to seeing what is actually there. If we can bring the fresh eyes of a beginner or child to our experience, we discover all kinds of things. We can apply this to sleep by approaching each night free of the expectations or emotions that are the result of the previous night.

# Keeping a sleep diary

It's useful to keep a note of what you discover once you start paying attention to your routine and behavior and noticing how that affects your sleep, whether positively or negatively.

You might want to note what is happening for you at work or home, if you are working extra hours or doing shift work, and if you are traveling, particularly across time zones. It's fine to estimate times and amounts for awakenings and activities, and for food and drink consumption. Note any insights into what may be helping or hindering your sleep. If you start implementing new positive habits, make a note of what they are and what you notice. Small changes make a difference, so alter one thing at a time and continue it for at least a couple of weeks.

The aim of the sleep diary is to give you an insight into what you could do to help yourself. Generally, when we become aware of unhelpful habits, we naturally begin to change them. However, it is important not to become fixated on doing things in a particular way. If you find that keeping notes increases your anxiety, perhaps set them aside for a while. Practicing mindfulness encourages flexibility and a willingness to be with the way things are, so in time you may find it helpful to go back to trying a sleep diary if you would like to.

## Remember to be gentle on yourself

There's no need to be critical of anything you notice; simply notice cause and effect. If you have a day when you slip back into unhelpful habits, just notice how they affect your sleep, rather than giving yourself a hard time. Noticing how you talk to yourself when things don't go to plan, and practicing self-compassion, is as much a mindfulness practice as meditating for 15 minutes. Change takes time and it's rarely linear—there will be good days and nights, and those that are less good. When you experience the latter, it doesn't mean that everything you have been doing has been worthless. It's just the way things are.

Work on the sleep diary for a specific period of time (at least 2 weeks) so that you can build up a picture of which habits are helpful for you and which are not. Once you are familiar with which habits are helpful for you and which aren't, let go of the need to record how much sleep you have had or not. It's similar to the way weighing ourselves every day can be counterproductive, since we often start obsessing about

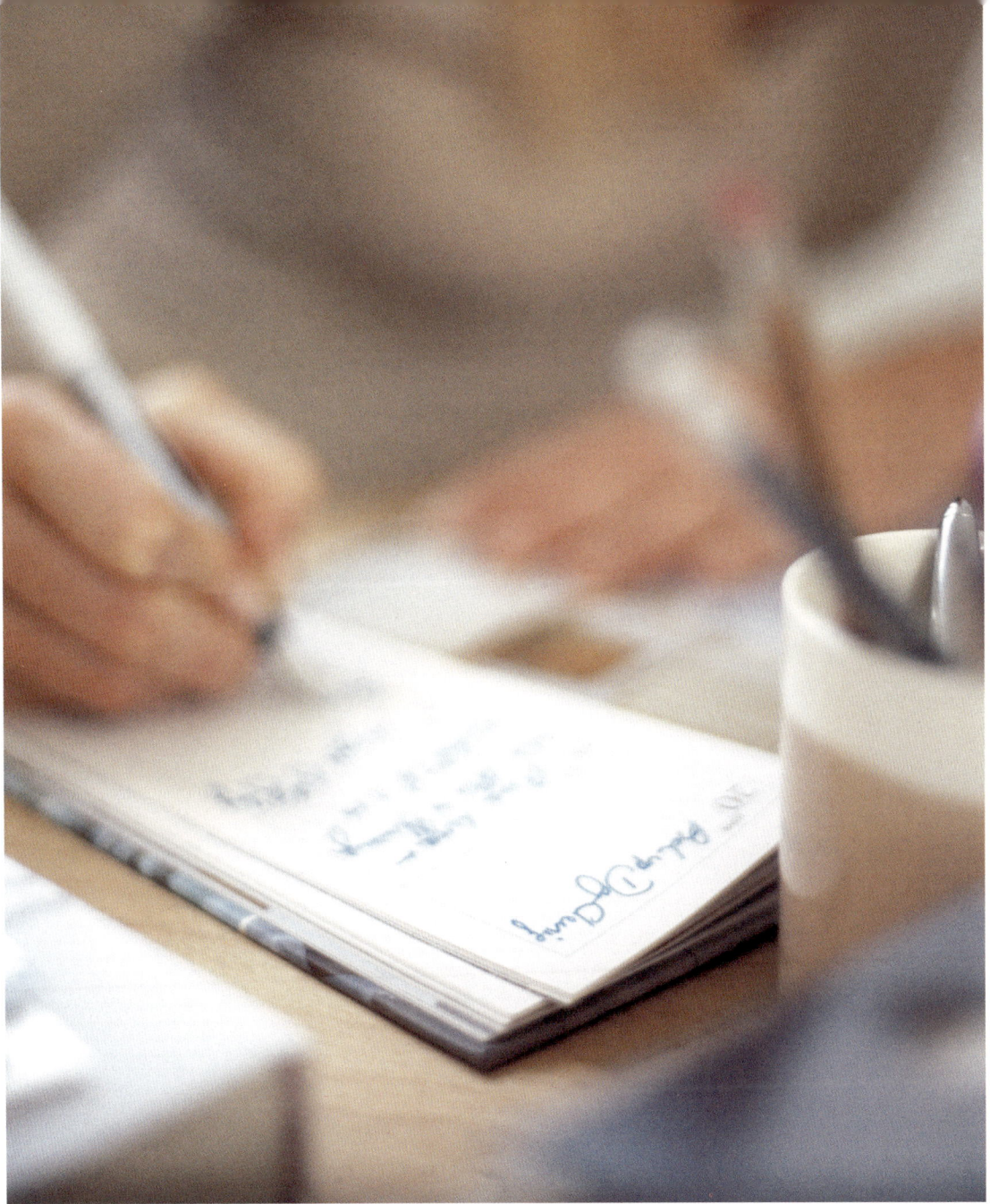

minor changes up and down. The less anxious we are about how much sleep we are getting, the more likely we are to feel more relaxed—and that is conducive to feeling rested and refreshed and possibly sleeping better.

# CBD for relaxation

Using CBD (cannabidiol) can aid relaxation, especially when it is paired with essential oils (see page 94). Unlike THC (tetrahydrocannabinol), the psychoactive chemical element of cannabis and hemp plants, you can benefit from the therapeutic effects of CBD without any psychedelic effects.

CBD is what we call a cannabinoid. Cannabinoids are chemical compounds found in the cannabis plant. They closely resemble compounds called endocannabinoids that our own bodies produce naturally. It is considered to be one of the most effective compounds to help support our immune system and decrease anxiety and depression, as well as being an influential neuroprotectant, defending and supporting the vital neurons that make up our brain function.

Two major contributors to the breakdown of brain cells are oxidation and inflammation, and CBD has very robust antioxidant and anti-inflammatory properties. It also acts as an anticonvulsant, antipsychotic, anti-anxiety, analgesic, antidepressant, and neuroprotective natural plant compound. Many of these properties happen to be immensely helpful for skincare conditions, too, including aging, dehydration, dullness, blotchiness, acne, psoriasis, eczema, and excessive pigmentation.

## The science behind it

When CBD is absorbed by our skin, it makes its way to our endocannabinoid system (abbreviated as ECS) and stimulates it. The endocannabinoid system is a remarkable network of compounds and receptors in the brain often described as a central component of the health and healing of every human and almost every animal. This vast grid has the capacity to influence functions in the brain, including memory, mood, pain response, appetite, perception, cognition, sleep, emotions, motor function, and anti-inflammatory function, as well as brain development and protection.

The ECS is omnipresent in the body—in the skin, the brain, major organs, connective tissue, glands, immune cells, etc. In each area of the body, it carries out different tasks, but the goal is always the same and it is a rather wonderful one: the ECS works tirelessly to maintain the body's internal balance and physical wellbeing. It creates an internal equilibrium, harmony, and peace, which resists even the most hostile fluctuations in the external environment.

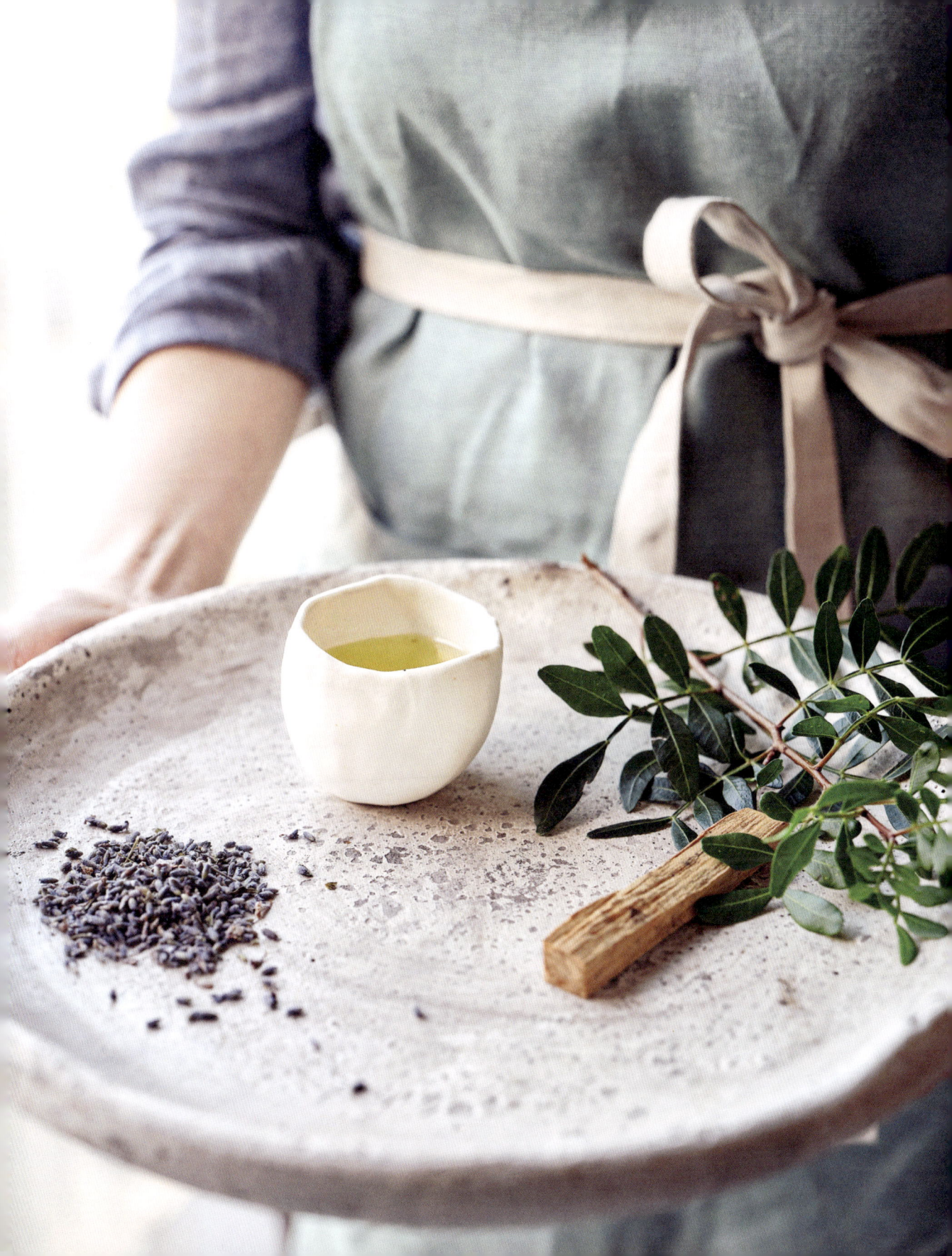

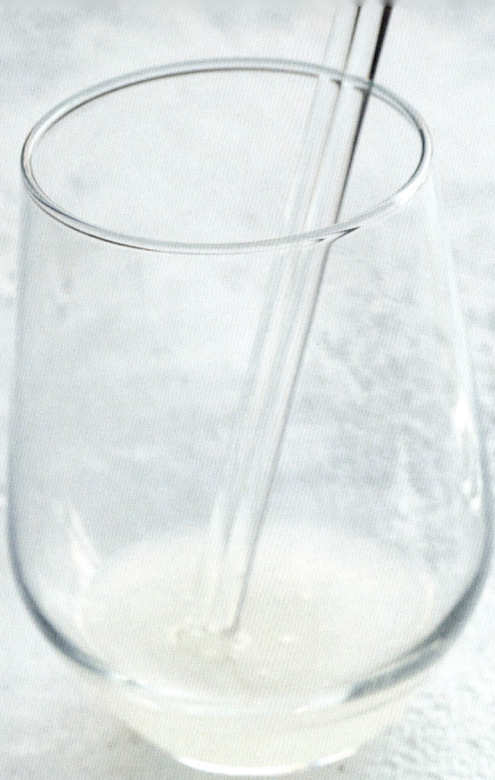

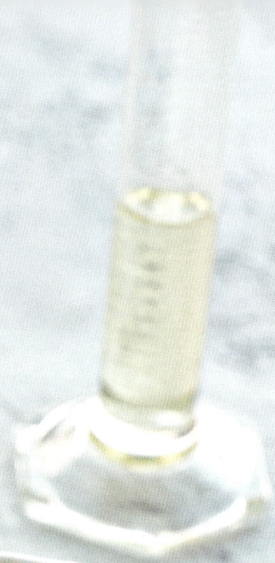

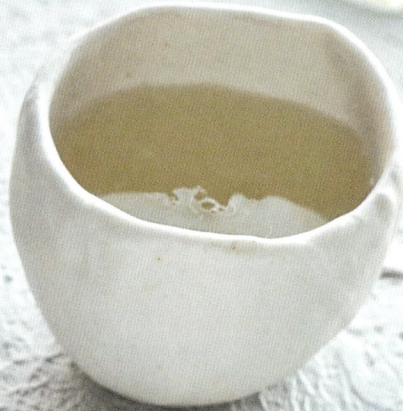

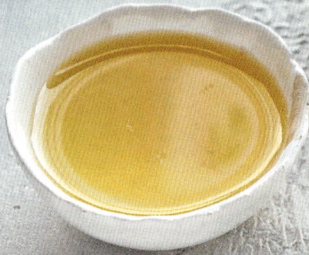

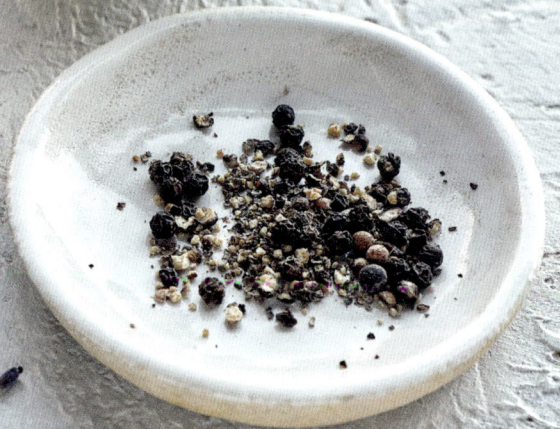

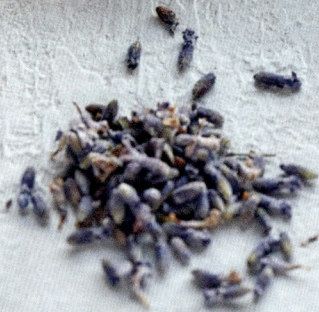

# HOW TO CHOOSE A CBD OIL

There are so many CBD products on the market today that you can get tricked into buying something that isn't the real deal. Follow these guidelines to help you choose.

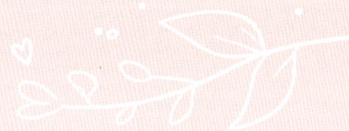

## Legal considerations

Be sure you are familiar with the cannabis legislation where you live.

## Use a reputable brand

When buying your CBD oil, it is important to choose reputable brands with a history of supplying plant-based concentrations.

## CBD content

It may sound obvious, but you do need to check that the product you are purchasing actually contains CBD! A lot of stores are selling hempseed carrier oil as cannabis or CBD oil, which it is not. You may also see a product called cannabis or hemp essential oil. It is important to understand that this admittedly lovely oil is not CBD oil. An "essential oil" is a distillation of plant material and this action captures the volatile components—for example, the aromatic terpenes. Cannabinoids are considered non-volatiles: they are fat-loving, not water-loving. This means that they cannot be distilled effectively and therefore cannot end up in the plant's essential oil.

## Label information

Look at the label. It should include:

- Concentration of CBD: While it's possible to use up to 10,000 mg of CBD oil per 1 fl oz (30 ml) in your recipes (such as those on pages 96–105), it's better to stick to a concentration of 300 mg of CBD oil per 1 fl oz (30 ml) for relaxing remedies.
- Batch number: You should be able to see a batch number on the label to ensure the product is traceable to the manufacturer in case of any problems with it.
- Best by date: This is vital so that you can gauge the freshness of the product and ensure you use it before it expires.

## Lab report/Certificate of Analysis

It is very important to look for a Certificate of Analysis (COA) for the product you are interested in. This should be readily available on the brand's website. It is important to know if the analysis was performed by an accredited laboratory. A good indication will be if they are accredited in accordance with the International Organization for Standardization (ISO). This report will show you the CBD concentration. It is a nice comfort check to ensure your product truly has the CBD concentration advertised. Note that the lab report should be reasonably recent, preferably within the last 12 months.

# Ways to use CBD

CBD products come in many different formats. One of the simplest ways to use CBD is by applying an infused oil, cream, or salve. You can find recipes to make at home on pages 96–105.

## TOPICAL APPLICATION

We know that topical CBD products interact with cannabinoid receptors in the skin and nervous system. Applying CBD oil to the skin works best when consistently applied directly to areas of chronic inflammation or pain, and if combined synergistically with other botanicals and essential oils (see page 94) to increase permeability. Another option is a transdermal patch. Transdermal delivery refers to a topical application that has been modified to increase absorption through the skin (in much the same way as a nicotine patch works).

## SMOKING OR VAPING

Traditionally, smoking was the most common way of consuming the plant. Today, cannabis flower or concentrate is often inhaled using a vape pen. Whether smoking or vaping, the cannabinoids are delivered directly to the blood and brain via the lungs. Terpenes are also volatilized and delivered directly to the brain through the same process. The effects of inhaled cannabinoids are experienced intensely and almost immediately.

## ORAL CONSUMPTION

When cannabis is consumed orally, it has a very different effect compared to when it is smoked. It can take up to two hours to enter the bloodstream. However, once in the bloodstream, it tends to stay there for much longer than smoked cannabis—sometimes up to four to six hours, as opposed to only two hours when smoked. Orally consumed cannabis has a more potent effect and a longer duration, making it a great choice for nighttime use, particularly in cases of chronic pain-related insomnia.

Many oral CBD products are available as alcohol-based tinctures or edibles like gummies, chocolate, or candy. As with all orally consumed cannabis, there is a risk of taking too much and having an unpleasant experience. Since it can take up to two hours to feel the effects, you might be tempted to take an additional amount. If one's ideal dose is exceeded in this way, there can be an increase in side-effects, including anxiety, paranoia, sleepiness, tachycardia (a heartbeat exceeding the normal rate), and even mild hallucinations.

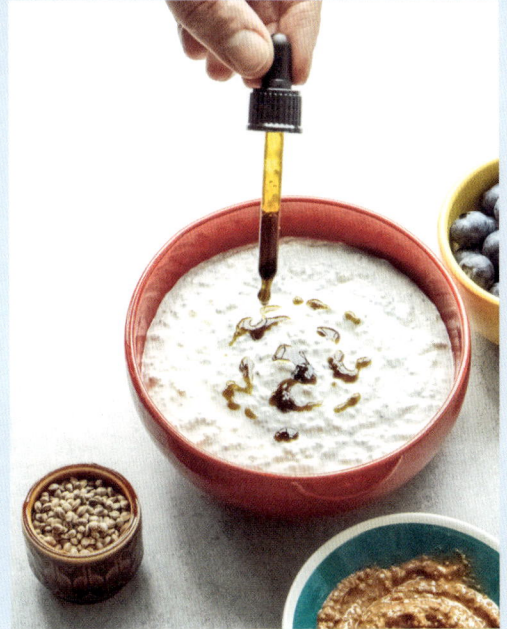

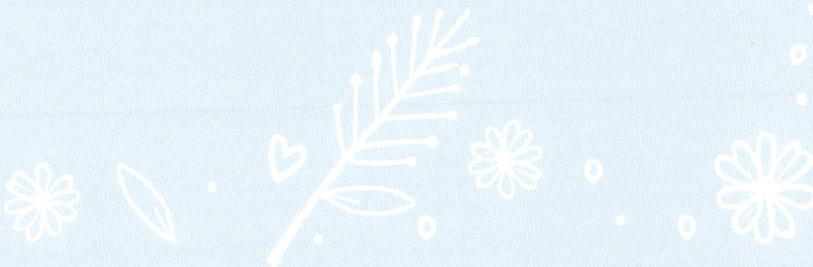

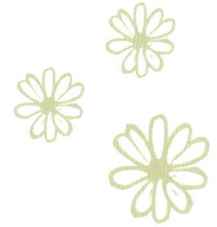

# The power of essential oils

Essential oils are the distilled aromatic essence of a plant. They are made by steaming or cold-pressing various parts of a plant (flowers, bark, leaves, or fruit) to capture the compounds that produce fragrance.

Plants are packed with phytochemicals—a powerful group of nutritive and antioxidant compounds that also provide plants with their color, flavor, and aroma. Each essential oil consists of hundreds of these phytochemicals. Essential oils are unique in so many ways, even down to their color, their viscosity, and the amount of plant material required to make the oils. You would need 60 roses to acquire one drop of rose essential oil, whereas the rind of five lemons will yield 20 drops of lemon essential oil.

## The science behind it

The sense of smell is the most primal of our senses. When essential oils are inhaled, they go directly to the brain and the impact of their therapeutic properties is almost immediate. For example, if we inhale an essential oil with sedating properties, such as ylang-ylang, it will produce a relaxing response very rapidly.

Essential oils can strengthen and calm your mind, nourish your soul, stimulate sensuality, support your immunity, love your skin, heal your body, and balance your mood. Their range and versatility are breathtaking. A single oil is also a multitasker most of the time. Lavender essential oil can relieve skin irritation, soothe muscular discomfort, and calm nervous tension in one application. Rosemary will act simultaneously to clear blocked sinuses, stimulate hair growth, gently settle nervous anxiety, and promote mental clarity and focus.

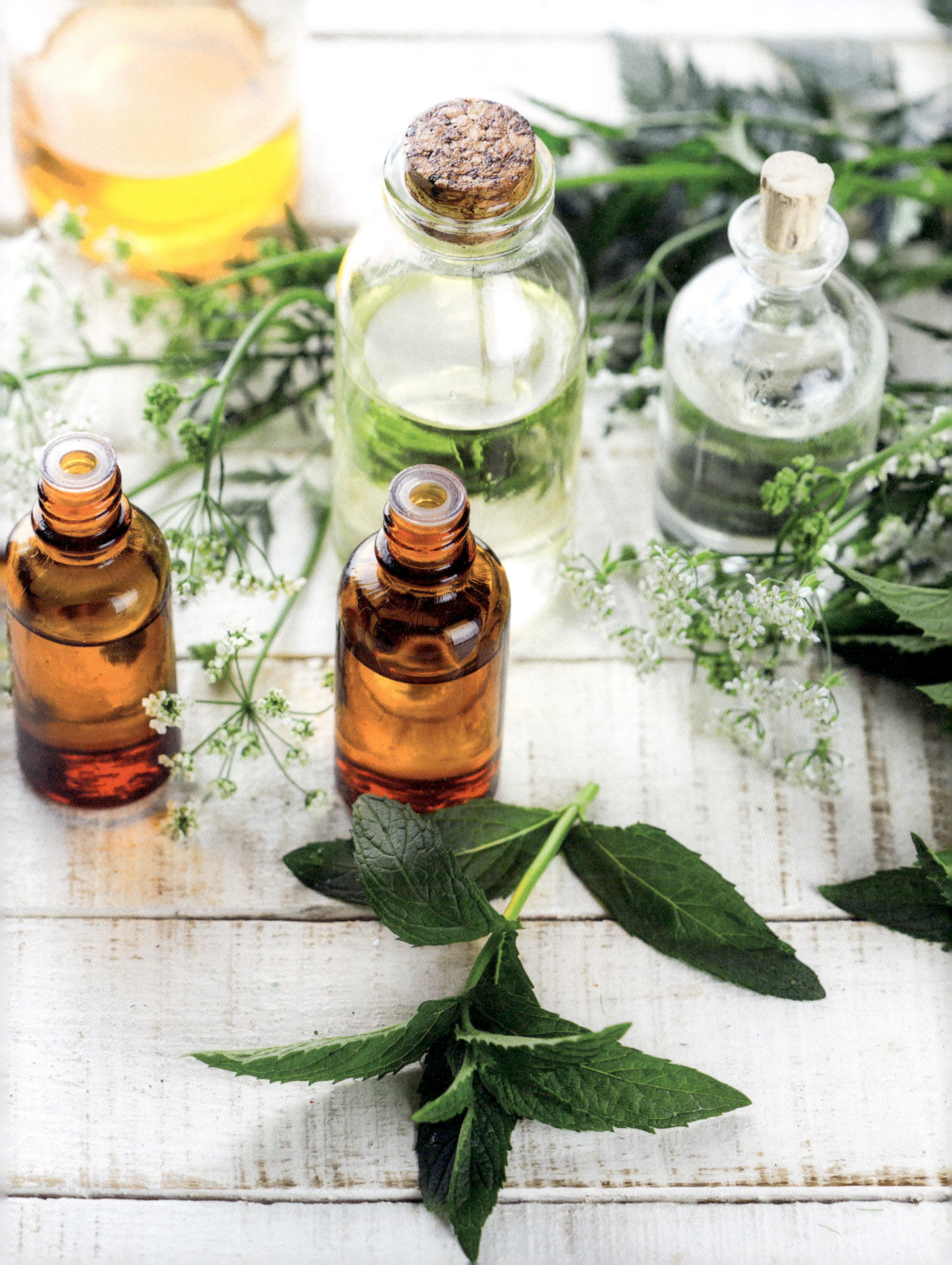

# Relaxation recipes

Discover how to use natural ingredients, combining CBD oil and essential oils, to aid rest and sleep.

When making your own recipes, you should use a separate set of bowls and beakers, as many of the ingredients, especially CBD oil, essential oils, and botanical ingredients, will leave a taste on your equipment that you will not want to impart to food.

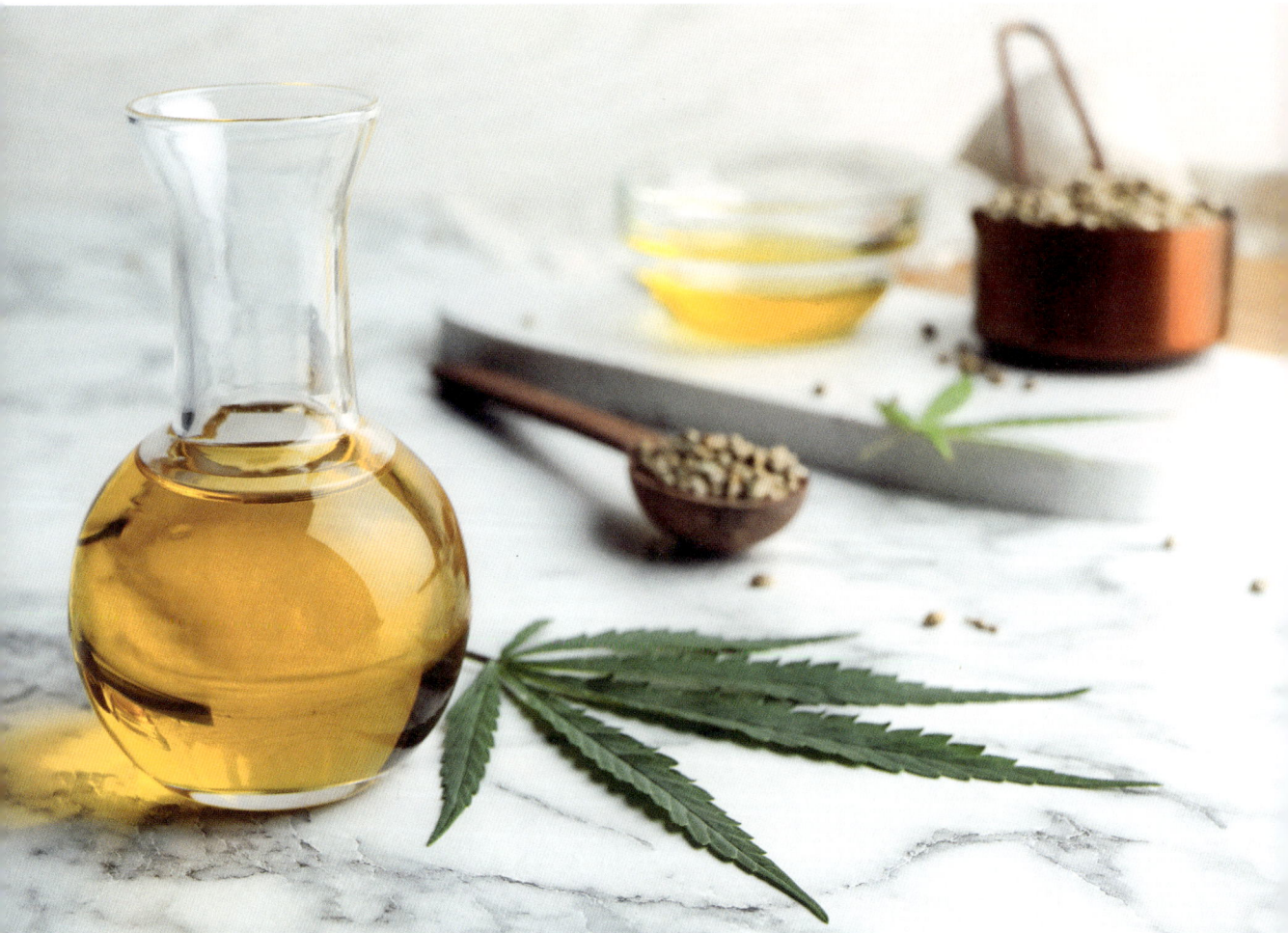

# FRANKINCENSE NOURISHING BODY OIL

2 tablespoons olive oil

1 tablespoon hempseed oil

1 teaspoon peach kernel oil

1 teaspoon CBD oil

10 drops cedarwood essential oil

6 drops frankincense essential oil

3 drops orange essential oil

## EQUIPMENT

Glass or stainless-steel beaker

Glass or wooden stirrer

2-fl oz (60-ml) glass bottle with dropper cap or flip lid

*Makes: 2 fl oz (60 ml)*

Frankincense has been used since the most ancient times for medicinal and wellness purposes. It was considered more valuable than gold and was burned as an offering to the gods. Its fragrance promotes feelings of calm, relaxation, and wellbeing, and in the beauty world the oil is prized for its ability to regenerate and rejuvenate the skin. This recipe partners frankincense with vitamin E-rich peach kernel oil and hempseed oil, which is brimming with omega-3, -6, and -9.

Combine the olive, hempseed, peach kernel, and CBD oils in the beaker. Gently stir in the cedarwood, frankincense, and orange essential oils. Transfer the mixture to the glass bottle and seal.

**Storage:** As there is no water in this body oil, it will keep for up to three months if stored away from direct sunlight and heat.

**To use:** Generously massage into your skin after your daily shower or bath. The frankincense is the perfect resinous aroma to float through your senses just before bed.

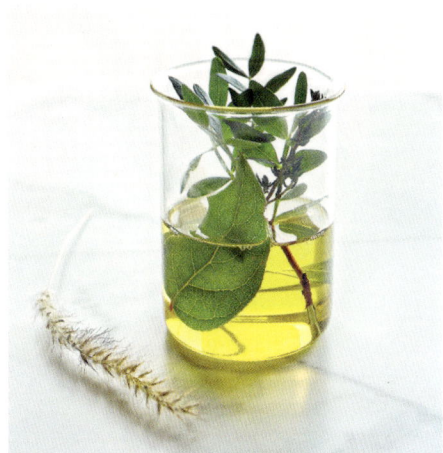

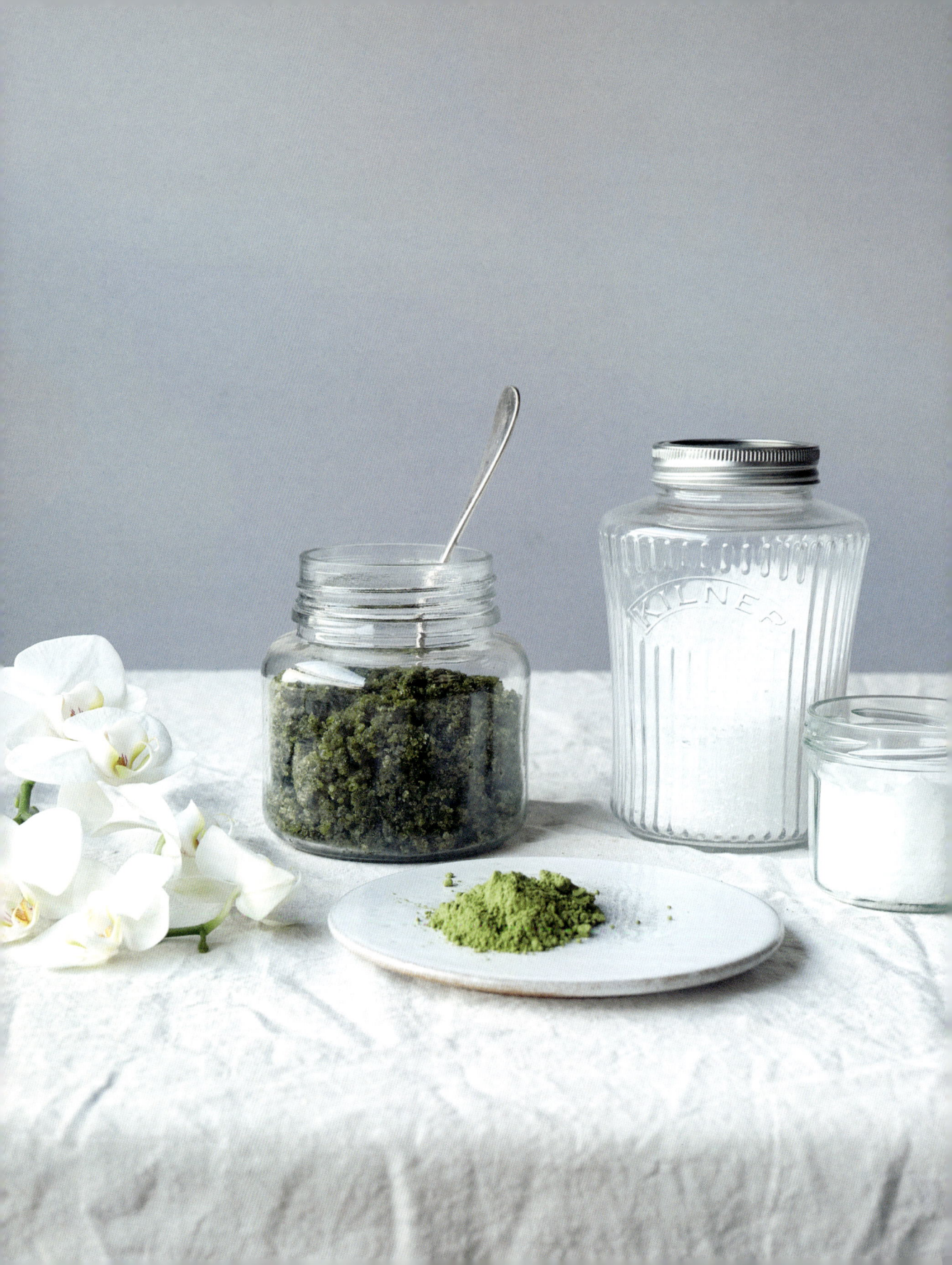

# MUSCLE-SOOTHING BATH SALTS

6 oz (170 g) Epsom salts

6 oz (170 g) magnesium flakes

3 oz (85 g) Dead Sea salts

1 tablespoon matcha powder

1 tablespoon CBD oil

20 drops rosemary
essential oil

20 drops frankincense
essential oil

20 drops cedarwood
essential oil

## EQUIPMENT

Glass or stainless-steel bowl

Glass or wooden stirrer

1-lb (450-g) glass jar with lid

*Makes: 1 lb (450 g)*

Boost CBD oil's analgesic and anti-inflammatory properties with magnesium flakes and Epsom salts. Low magnesium intake is linked to chronic inflammation, which is a major source of pain and one of the drivers of aging. Interestingly, one of the most effective ways of absorbing magnesium is through your skin rather than via your digestive system—so a therapeutic soak is thoroughly recommended for those tired and sore muscles!

Combine the Epsom salts, magnesium flakes, and Dead Sea salts in the bowl. Add the matcha powder and stir until the entire mixture turns a shade of light green. Stir in the CBD oil and rosemary, frankincense, and cedarwood essential oils. Transfer the mixture to the glass jar and seal.

**Storage:** This large jar will last up to four months. Keep it sealed when not in use to avoid moisture getting into the salts.

**To use:** Scoop two heaped tablespoons of the muscle-soothing salts into the bathtub as you run the water. Add a little extra if your body is tired or if you have been overworking those muscles. Be sure to use a non-slip bathmat.

**Note:** Make sure to clean your bathtub well immediately after use, as the matcha can be difficult to remove once it dries.

# ROSE PETAL VEGAN BATH MILK

5½ oz (150 g)
chickpea flour

Vanilla pod

Handful of rose petals, fresh
or dried

2 oz (55 g) cocoa
butter, chilled

3 teaspoons CBD oil

10 drops geranium
essential oil

10 drops ylang-ylang
essential oil

## EQUIPMENT

Glass or stainless-steel bowl

Standard kitchen grater

Glass or wooden stirrer

8-oz (225-g) glass jar with lid

*Makes: 1 lb (450 g)*

A bath is one of the greatest gifts we can give ourselves and adding some therapeutic and aromatic ingredients to that bath is obligatory. This recipe is a vegan alternative to dairy. With its cocoa butter, CBD oil, and heavenly geranium and ylang-ylang essential oils, it is no less luxurious and emollient.

Combine the chickpea flour, vanilla pod, and rose petals in the bowl. Grate the chilled cocoa butter into the bowl. Stir in the CBD oil and the geranium and ylang-ylang essential oils. Transfer to the glass jar and seal.

**Storage:** This recipe will keep for up to a year unopened, but use it up within six weeks once the seal is broken. The longer you leave this bath milk sealed in the jar, the more aromatically infused the mixture will become. The fragrant scent from the jar once you open it will be stunningly beautiful and the bathing experience is one of the most luxurious you will ever have.

**To use:** While you are running your bath, add three scoops of the bath milk. Swirl it around with your hand to ensure even distribution. If you are feeling very Cleopatra-like, add an additional scoop for a milkier bath! Be sure to use a non-slip bathmat.

**Note:** Never heard of chickpea flour and certainly never in a skincare recipe? Don't worry—it is not a crazy concept! Chickpea flour will soothe and smooth your skin, leaving you emerging from your bath with baby-soft skin.

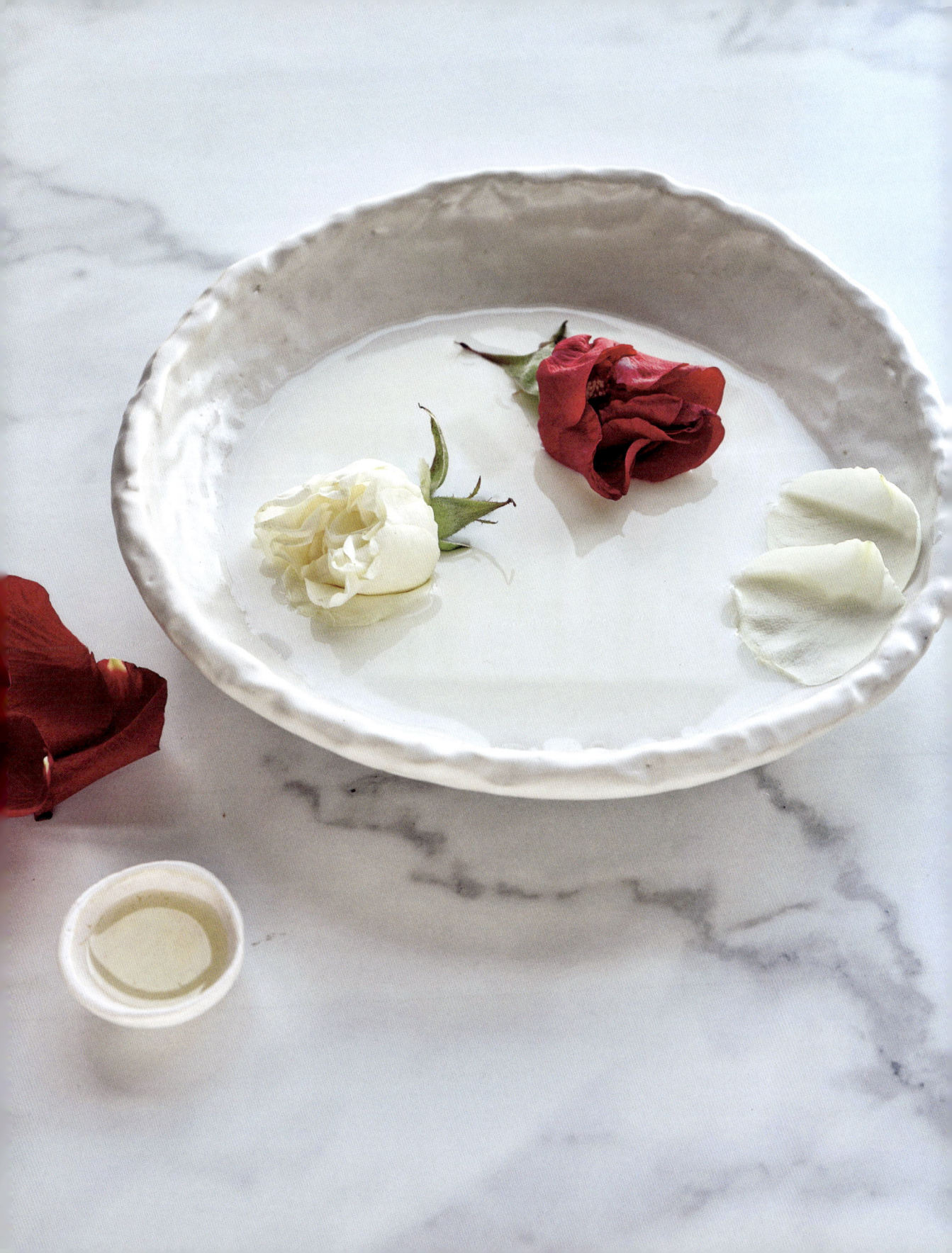

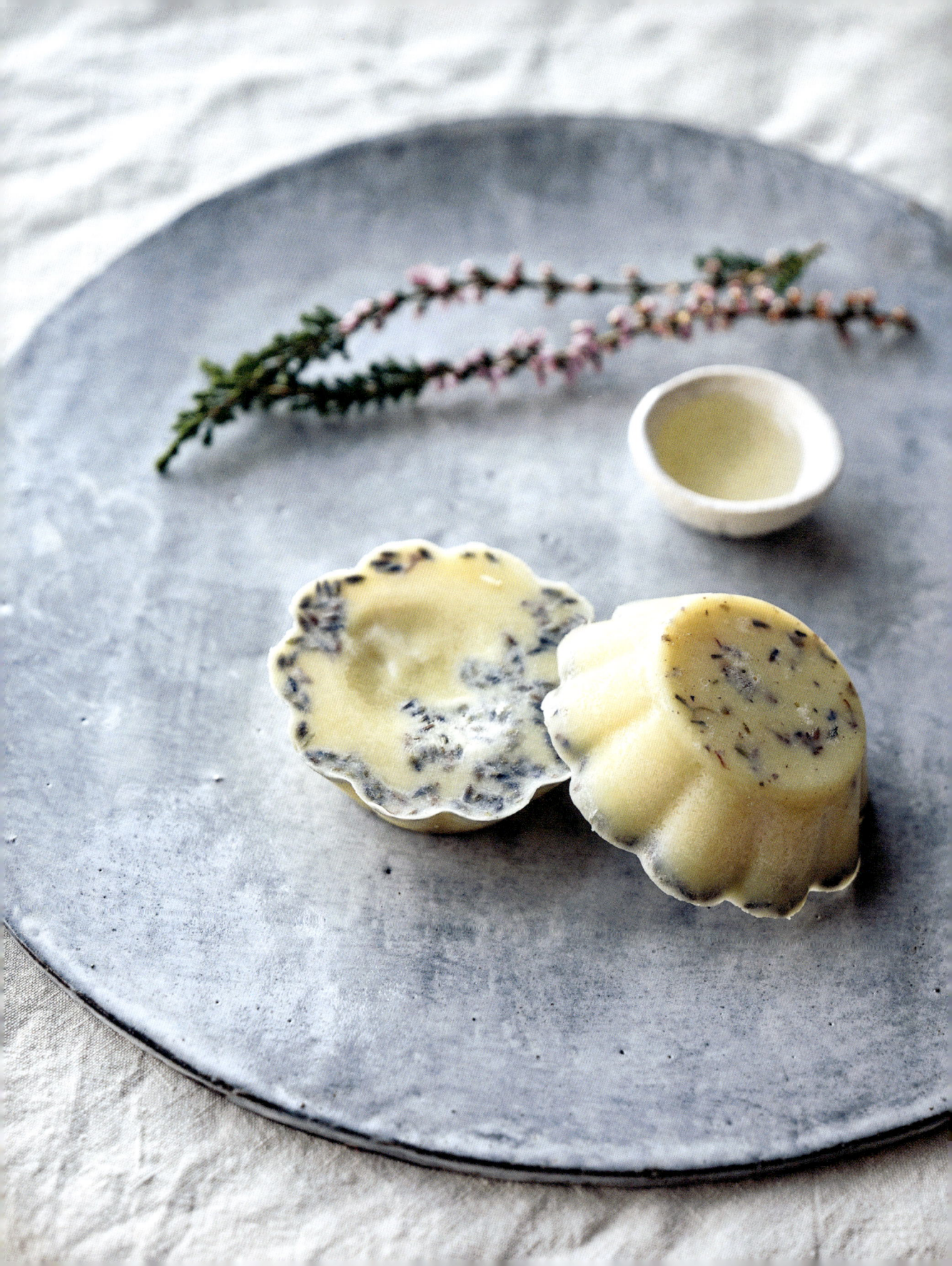

# LAVENDER SLEEP MASSAGE BAR

1 oz (30 g) cocoa butter

½ oz (15 g) shea butter

1 teaspoon CBD oil

10 drops lavender essential oil

10 drops cedarwood essential oil

10 drops frankincense essential oil

1 teaspoon dried lavender flowers

## EQUIPMENT

Double boiler

Stainless-steel bowl

Glass stirrer

2 x 1-oz (30-g) molds or 6 smaller paper muffin/cupcake cases

*Makes: two 1-oz (30-g) molds, but this recipe can yield up to six small bars if you choose to use small bun cases instead of larger molds*

Lavender has long been the go-to essential oil for promoting restful sleep. Here it is joined by CBD oil to form a highly effective sleep support. Pain, stress, and anxiety are three of the major causes of sleep disturbance, and CBD oil works effectively on all three fronts. Blending these formidable sleep aids in one recipe creates a truly blissful tool for encouraging a peaceful night between the sheets.

Melt the cocoa butter and shea butter in the double boiler. Remove the mixture from the heat and gently stir in the CBD oil and lavender, cedarwood, and frankincense essential oils, followed by the lavender flowers. Pour the mixture into the molds and place in the refrigerator to set for one to two hours. Once the mixture has set, peel the massage bars from the molds.

**Storage:** The massage bars will keep for up to a year if stored somewhere cool.

**To use:** Massage into the body as needed, before going to sleep.

**Note:** The base of shea and cocoa butters in these massage bars allows a smooth massage application. They nourish and condition as you work the aromatic sleep-inducing plant nutrients into your skin.

# AROMATHERAPY BATH TEABAGS

2 tablespoons Dead Sea salts

1 tablespoon dried
lavender flowers

1 tablespoon dried rose petals

1 tablespoon dried
nettle herb

1 tablespoon dried seaweed

1 teaspoon CBD oil

10 drops lavender essential oil

## EQUIPMENT

Glass or stainless-steel bowl

Glass or wooden stirrer

4 x 8-in. (20-cm) squares
of muslin

4 elastic bands

4 lengths of string or ribbon

*Makes: four teabags*

Herbal bath soaks are wonderfully relaxing. However, they can be very messy. The answer is to make your own bath "teabags" using muslin squares. That way, you have all the benefits of the herbs with none of the debris on your skin and bathtub.

Combine the Dead Sea salts, lavender flowers, rose petals, nettle herb, and seaweed in the bowl. Stir in the CBD oil and lavender essential oil. Spoon the mixture evenly into the four muslin squares. Gather the corners of each muslin square and secure with an elastic band. Tie the teabags with string—or ribbon, to make them oh-so pretty.

**Storage:** The teabags will keep for up to 12 months.

**To use:** Place one teabag into your bathtub and relax.

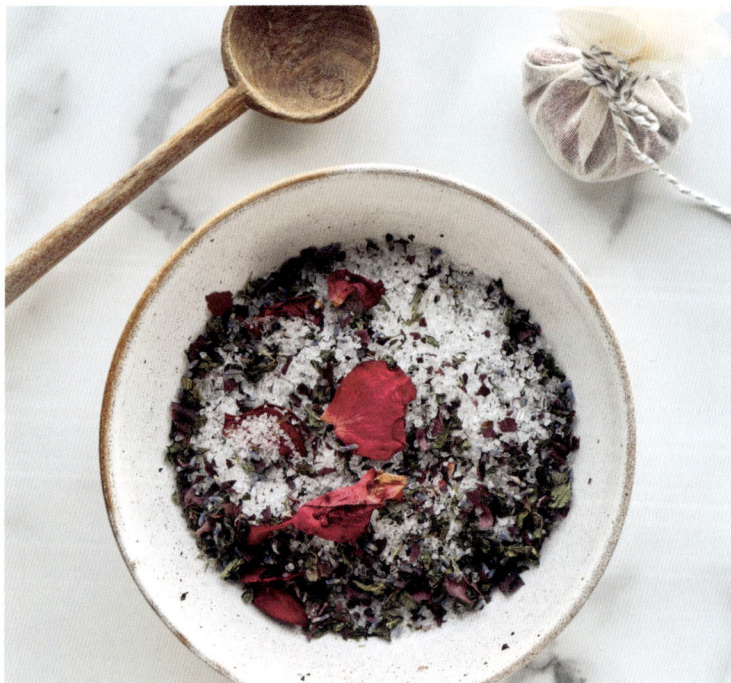

# RELAXING PILLOW SPRAY

4 teaspoons lavender hydrosol

1 teaspoon glycerine

1 teaspoon CBD oil

2 drops lavender essential oil

## EQUIPMENT

Glass or stainless-steel beaker

Glass or wooden stirrer

1-fl oz (30-ml) glass bottle
with spray application top

*Makes: 1 fl oz (30 ml)*

Infuse your pillow with heavenly lavender and relaxing CBD oil to ensure you have sweet, sweet dreams all night long!

Combine the lavender hydrosol, glycerine, and CBD oil in the beaker. Gently stir in the lavender essential oil. Transfer to the glass bottle and seal.

**Storage:** Store away from direct sunlight and heat. Your spray will stay fresh and aromatic for up to three weeks.

**To use:** Spray directly onto your pillow before sleep.

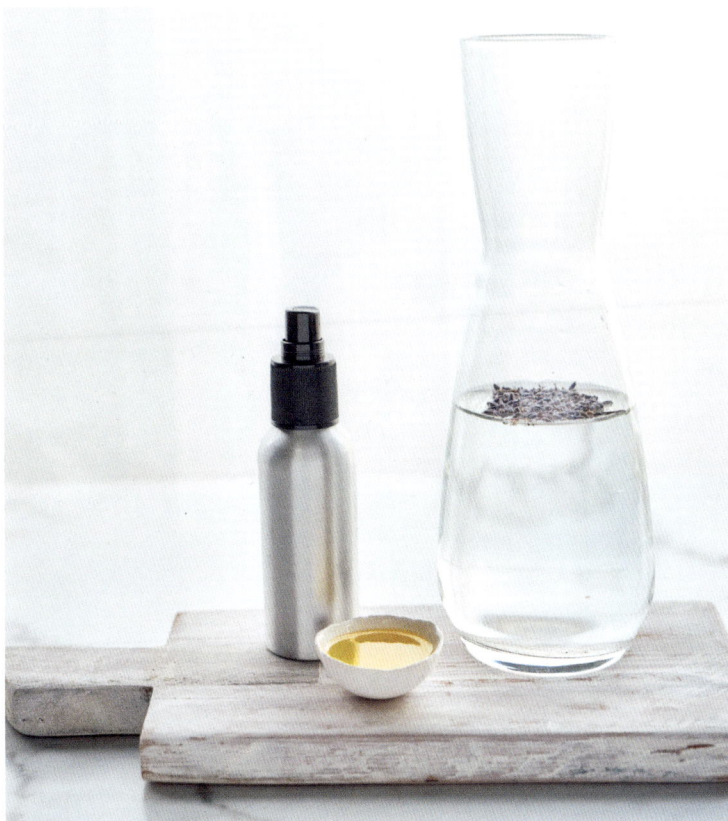

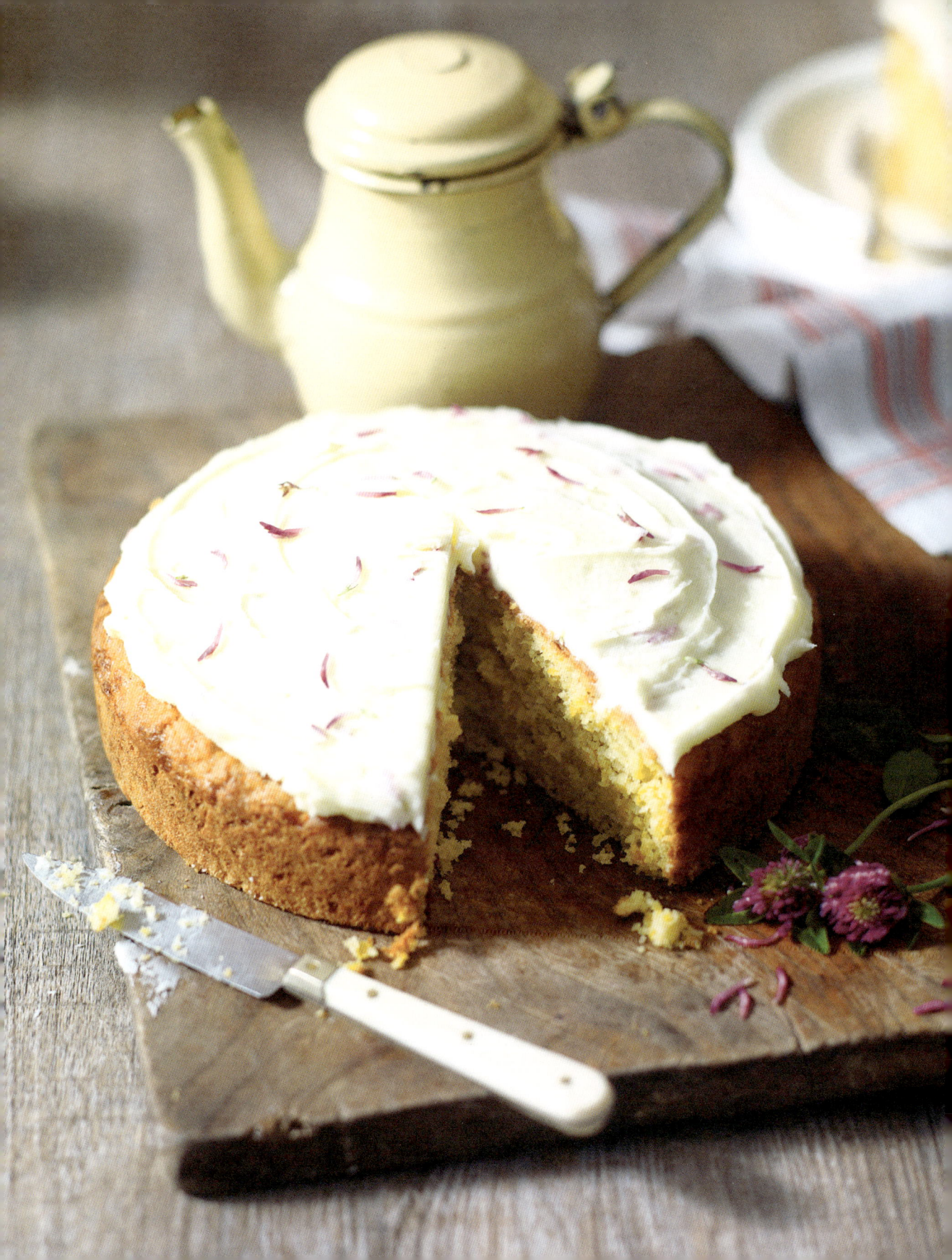

# Chapter 4

# *Finding* Happiness and *Joy*

Shift your thought patterns to unlock your potential, create positive change in your life, and achieve true happiness.

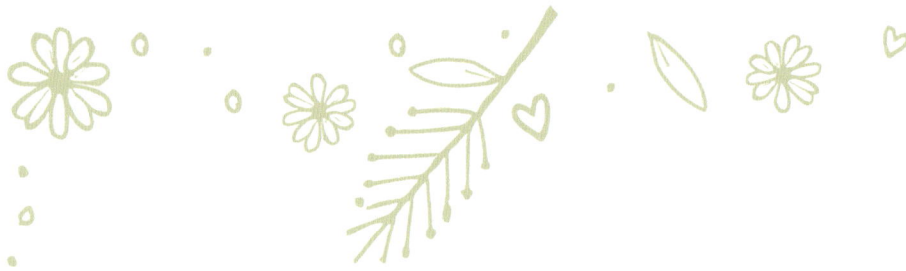

# Self-kindness is a strength

Many of us are more likely to practice meanness rather than kindness toward ourselves. We judge ourselves remorselessly, making unreasonable demands on ourselves and offering no quarter when we fall short. But we would never treat someone we cared about in this way.

Offering kindness toward ourselves is an invaluable practice and one that cannot be done too often, but it can take practice and self-discipline. If we do not practice it, we may cause harm to ourselves, as well as to others indirectly. Until we care for ourselves, and until we are at ease with who we are, we will not be at peace, and we will not be free to give all of our heart to others. If we are hard on ourselves, we allow our experiences to harden our hearts.

We all know people who seem to spend all their time giving to others and being friends to those around them, but who don't make time for themselves. If you are one of them, why not make a pledge to allow time for yourself and your needs? If you can't do it for yourself, do it for those who care about you, because the more you take care of your own sake, the more energy you will have to support the important people in your life. Book a haircut, decide to spend a weekend away, treat yourself to an afternoon off to read a book, listen to music, or go for a walk in nature. Get the bike out and head for the hills. Whatever you need to do to retune your senses and tune in to your inner self, now is the time to do it.

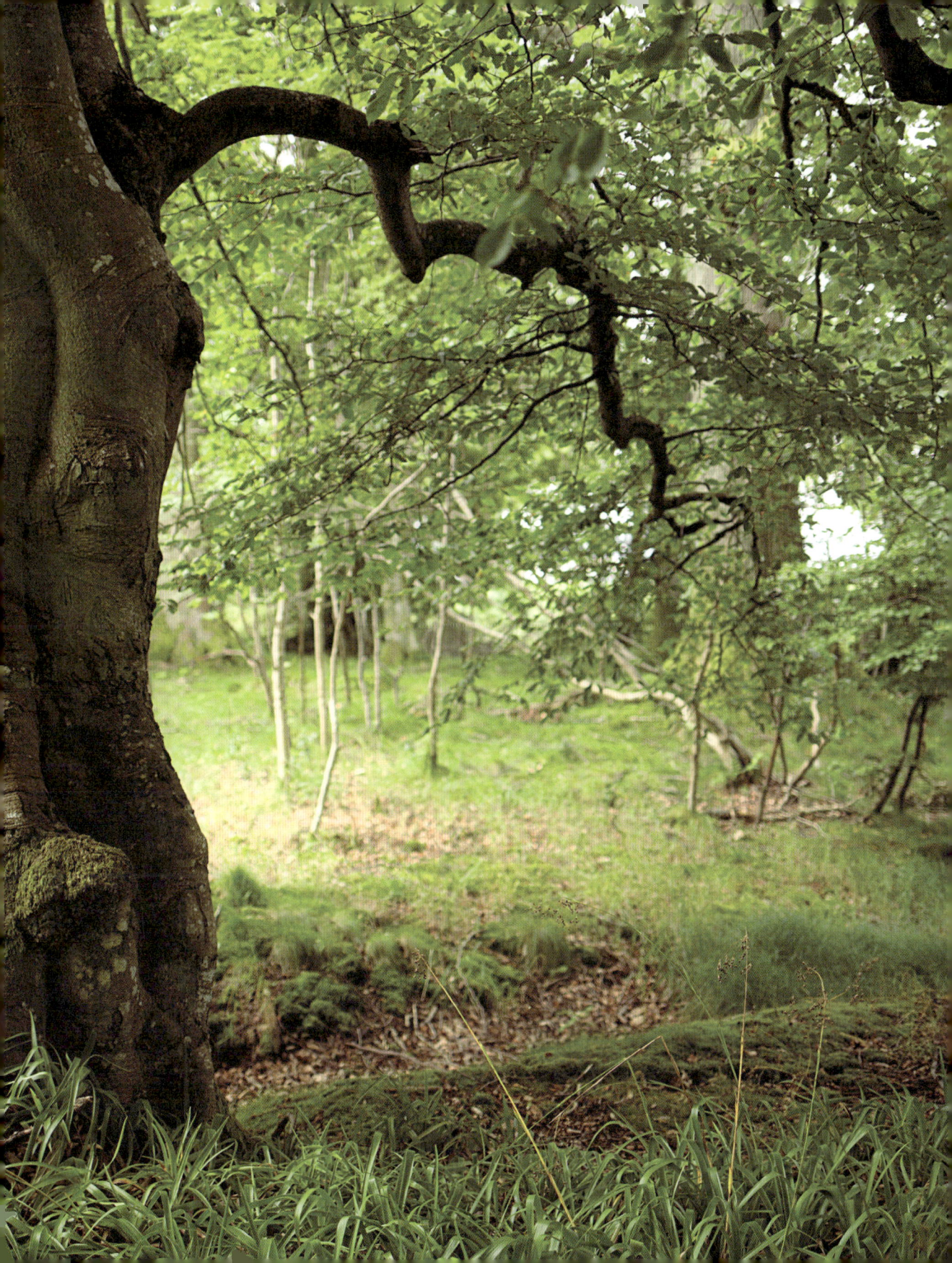

# Rediscover happiness for improved health

Scientists have finally proved it—happiness is good for you. Those who are happy or have an optimistic and positive outlook are far less likely to suffer from clinical depression. Happiness appears to lead to longer life, greater health, and increased levels of resilience.

Scientific study of the effects of happiness has an impressive pedigree. Aristotle pondered the causes and impact of happiness as long ago as 322 BC. He suggested that the pursuit of happiness was an essential part of being human, and a goal in itself.

More recently, scientists have discovered something that they call the "Happiness Paradox"—the more intent you are on pursuing solely your own path of happiness,

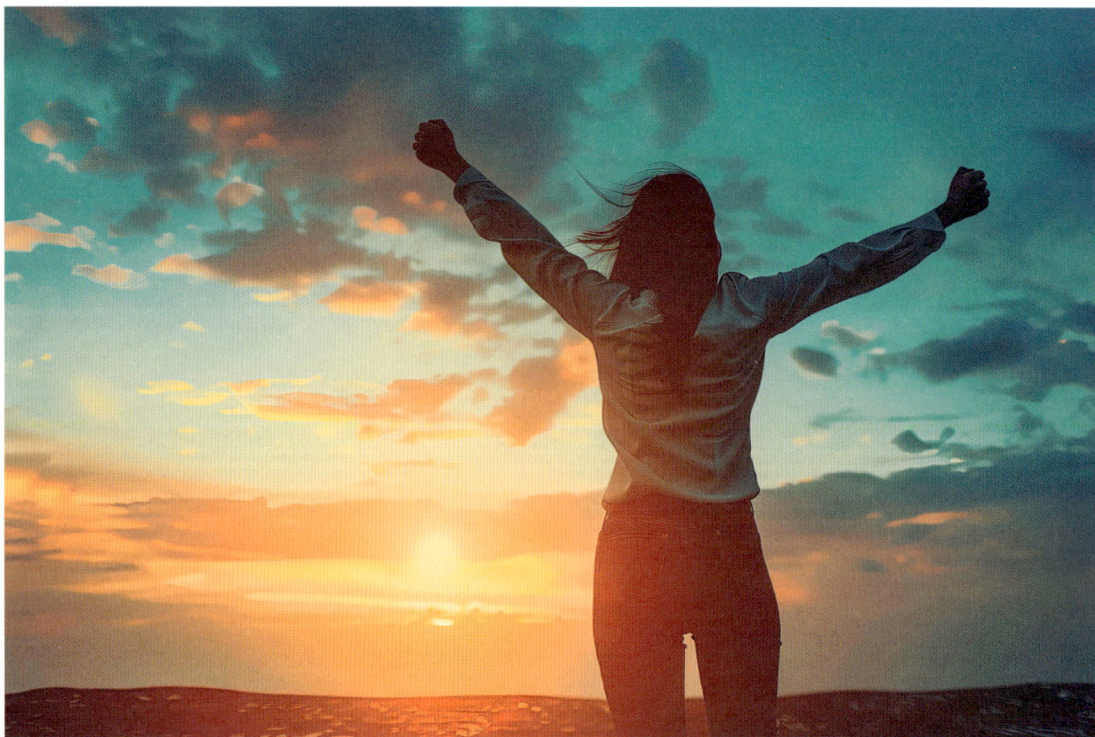

the less likely you are to feel happy; whereas the more willing you are to focus on and help other people with no thought of your own gain, the happier and more content you will be.

There is another paradox: even though the standard of living has increased in most western countries over the past 30 years, national levels of happiness have not increased at all.

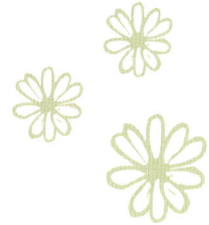

## The formula for happiness

In the early 1970s, 34 percent of people in the UK described themselves as "very happy." By the late 1990s, at a time when the country's economy was buoyant, the figure had dropped 4 percent. The improved standard of living across the country appeared to have had a slightly negative effect on the nation's happiness.

We are not quite as neighborly as we used to be, with 43 percent saying that neighbors are now less friendly than they were ten years ago, and only 22 percent saying their neighbors were more friendly now. But overall, we are a pretty contented bunch. A Happiness Formula poll found, in 2005, that 92 percent of people described themselves as either fairly happy or very happy. Only 8 percent said they were fairly or very unhappy; and over 60 percent spoke to up to five friends each week.

According to the 2025 World Happiness Report, the happiest country in the world is Finland, followed by Denmark, Iceland, Sweden, and the Netherlands. The United Kingdom is rated 23rd and the United States 24th.

On the one hand, the statistics are interesting and provide food for thought; they are the stuff of future government policies and social science surveys. On the other hand, it feels slightly absurd to think that happiness can be measured and verified. Surely there can be no completely reliable way to measure people's feelings?

It is encouraging to know that governments around the world are now setting policies that factor in the importance of happiness, but at the end of the day, no matter what the statistics say, each individual in every house, street, college and office has the power to determine the collective optimism of a nation as a whole.

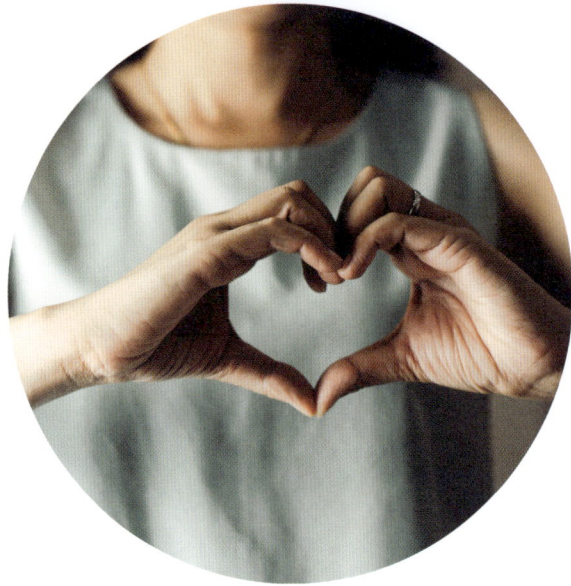

# Love reduces stress

One of the greatest obstacles to contentment is stress.
Of course, seeking a life without any stress is unrealistic,
but are there ways to manage and reduce it?

Scientists tell us that the roots of self-esteem stem from the earliest stages of our life. According to Sue Gerhardt, author of *Why Love Matters*, the unconditional love that we receive as babies appears to influence brain development. Babies who are comforted when they cry learn to soothe themselves as they grow; whereas babies who are left to cry develop a highly sensitized response to stress, which means that they find it harder to manage stress when they are adults.

But why is this? When we are stressed or feel in danger, the body produces a hormone called cortisol. We need a certain amount of cortisol, but in high-stress situations, we produce too much, too often, which can have a tiring effect on the body and leave people less able to manage their emotions. Those who are highly sensitive to stress will try to self-soothe—for example, by eating high-carbohydrate foods.

The good news is that getting physical with someone else will reduce your stress levels, reduce your cortisol levels, and increase the production of oxytocin, a "happy" hormone, in the body. All of this will make you feel happier, and will also boost your immune system.

## SIMPLE STRESS-BUSTERS

Don't worry about the science behind the results,
just make a mental note to:

- Hug a friend
- Get a massage
- Comfort a baby
- Hold hands with your loved one
- Stroke the dog
- Cuddle the cat
- Make love
- Go dancing
- Be more physical

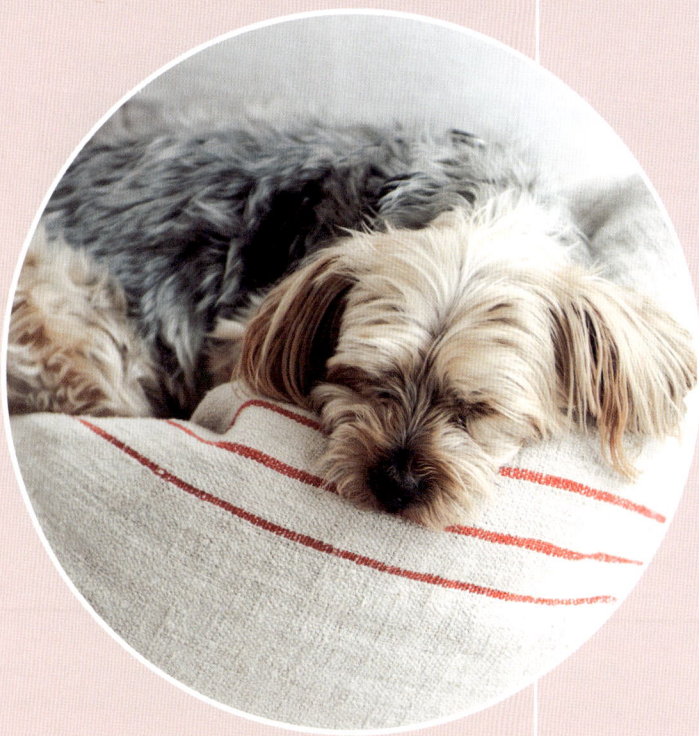

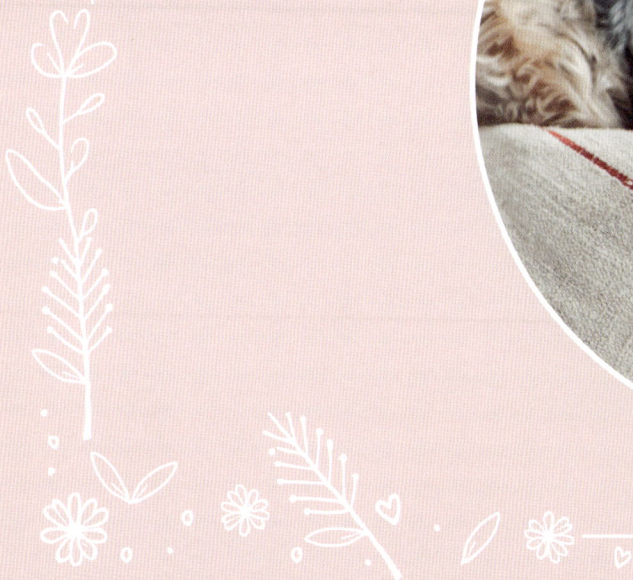

# Embrace spirituality

Many people lose their sense of happiness because they come to believe their life has no meaning. For many, this sense of loss stems from an absence of spiritual influence in their lives.

We are spiritual as well as physical beings, and can communicate by using our senses and mind—but in order to do so, we need to become aware of, and be back in tune with, our soul, as well as contemplate our place in the universe.

Scientists who have devoted their professional lives to understanding the nature of happiness, such as Martin Seligman, focus more on the mind than on the notion of the soul, but they have discovered that those who live a purposeful life are the happiest. A purposeful life tends to mean one that is focused on a goal or a mission that is greater than the needs of the individual. Altruism and selflessness enhance the chosen path. Great spiritual leaders, such as Mother Theresa, the Dalai Lama, and Archbishop Desmond Tutu, and more secular leaders, such as Nelson Mandela, Gandhi, and Aung San Suu Kyi, have all displayed a calm demeanor and a sense of purpose that give them a spiritual quality. They are acting for the greater good; the quest to improve the wellbeing of others has overtaken any inclination to focus solely on their own needs.

For many, spiritual awareness involves a ritual of worship. Prayers, chants, hymns, and offerings of thanks play an important role in every doctrine. The vibration, rhythm, and symbolism of each stage of the process have a profound effect on the human mind and body. These ancient ways make the body resonate, literally, with the power of the words and music. Those with greater understanding explain that it is by resonating at a higher level that it is possible to become in tune with the Divine.

Those who seek spiritual awareness are seekers after the ultimate truths in life; they are willing to give themselves over to a higher power and to have faith in life's greater purpose. Many on the path to spiritual happiness are searching for a state of bliss. Ironically, differences in spiritual doctrine and rigid adherence to the rules of religious dogma have been at the heart of wars, church schisms, civil unrest, and societies' prejudice for centuries. We seem no closer to universal peace and understanding now than at the time when religion began.

However, for the awakened soul, spirituality transcends dogma. Spirituality has little to do with the differences in the way we worship, and has everything to do with those aspects of our natures that are universal and that, at best, make human beings a force for good, and happiness epitomized.

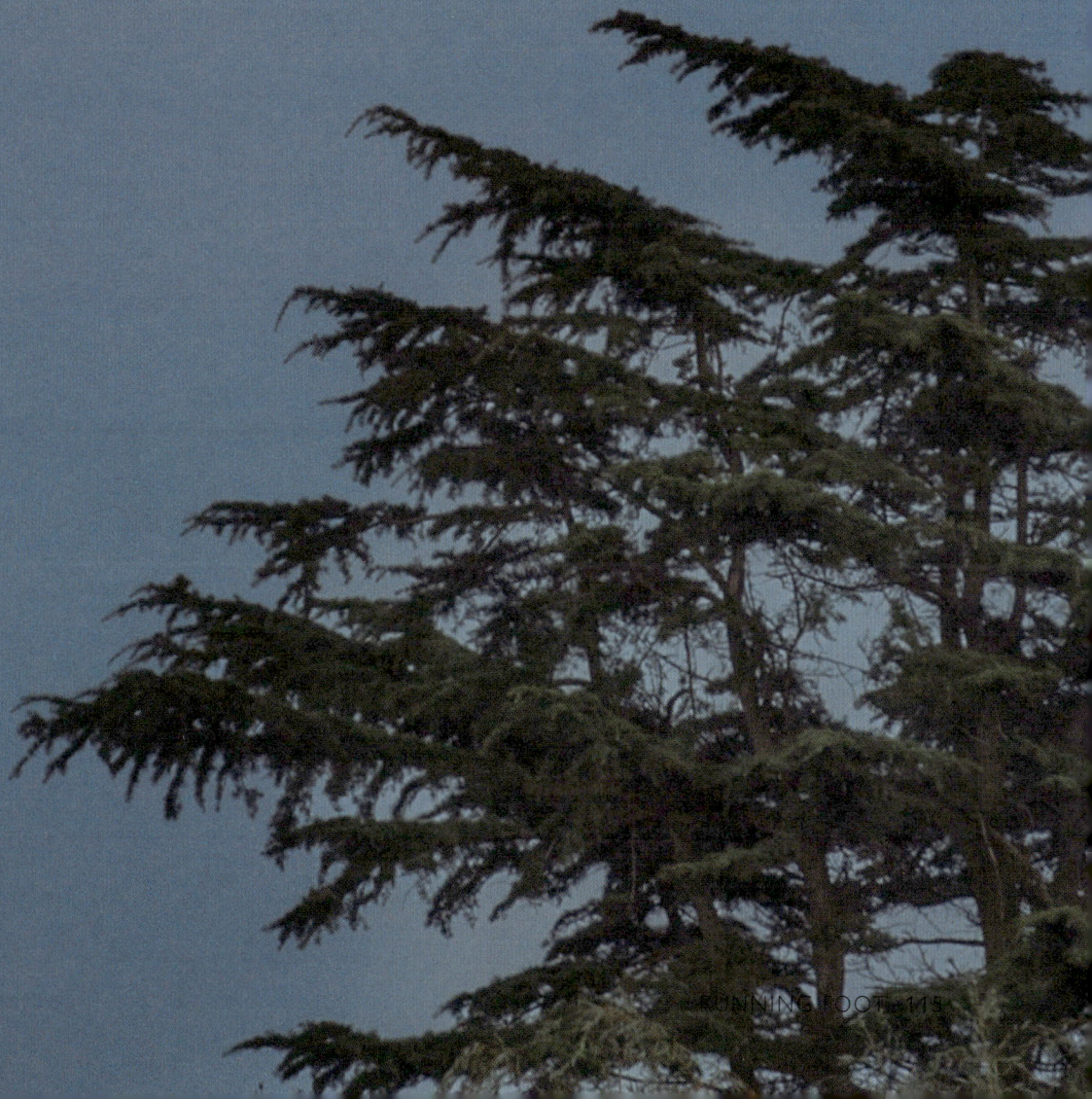

## ACHIEVING SPIRITUAL HAPPINESS

There are many and varied paths leading to spiritual awareness and everyone has to find their own way to meaning. Each religious tradition has its own set of belief systems and rituals, although at the heart of each doctrine the principles and basic practice are fundamentally the same:

- Belief in a higher power
- Faith
- Time devoted to learning about spiritual matters
- A general belief in our need to love one another as fellow human beings and to strive for a fairer and better world
- A ritual of prayer and devotion that has the power to make people feel closer to their higher power and stronger within themselves
- A call for a simple life, free of possessions and the trappings of materialism
- The teaching that we should love others more than ourselves

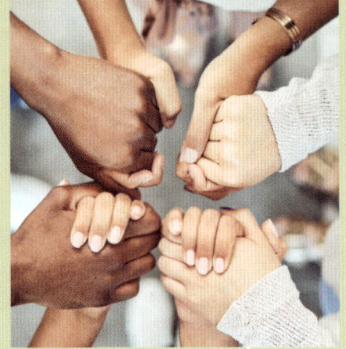

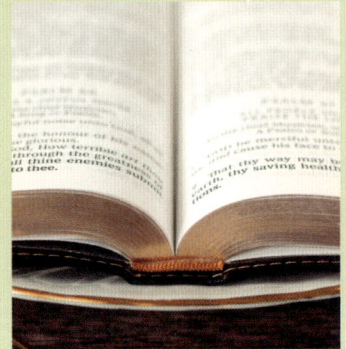

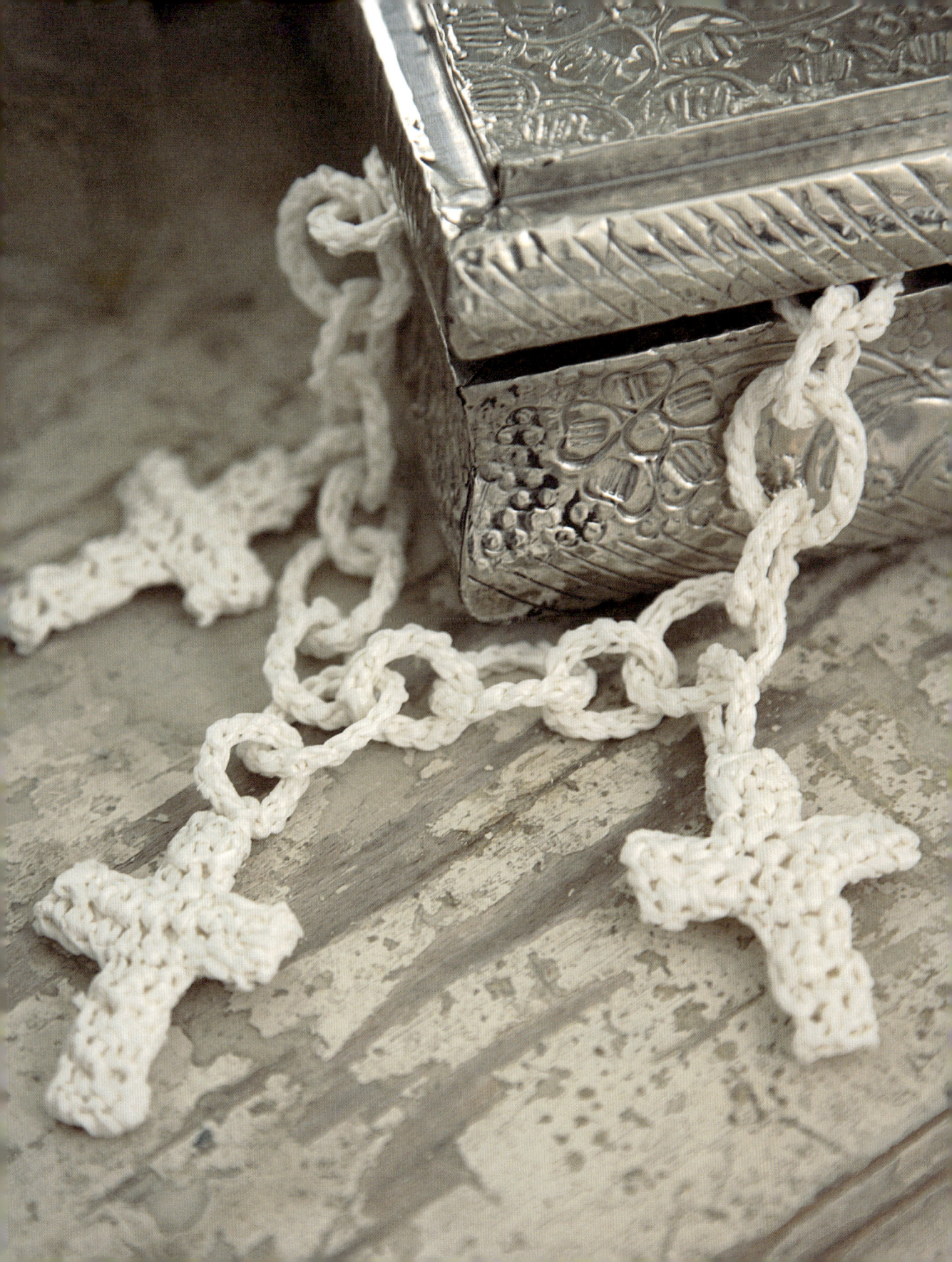

# Combat negativity

It is wise to try to immunize yourself against the power of negative thoughts before you are exposed to them, or to boost your levels of positive thinking if you know you have come into contact with them.

The symptoms of happiness are easy to spot and they are contagious. Children especially are liable to catch a bout of happiness very quickly and take great delight in passing it on. Cries of laughter, big smiles, the desire to run, jump, shout, and try new things are all symptomatic of the joyous impact of being happy. It may not last for very long, but it is powerful and fun while it lasts.

The symptoms of being less than happy are also contagious. They take hold more slowly, but may last for longer and show up in many ways. The common signs of chronic negativity are:

- **Reproachfulness.** You may blame yourself, your family, your job, your circumstances, for the way you are feeling about yourself and about your life.
- **Regret.** You may have a general sense of sadness; suffer feelings of worry and loneliness; feel unlovable, let down, or generally disappointed with life, your friends, or your achievements.
- **Anxiety.** You may feel overstretched, worried or worn down by responsibilities and the demands of others.
- **Self-defeating behavior.** You may be snappy and bad-tempered, feel a lack of personal motivation, and have a history of overeating, smoking, or drinking too much, or taking too little exercise; then feel sorry for yourself because of health problems or financial worries.
- **Becoming isolated.** Everyone has personal demons and self-destructive habits that jeopardize happiness from time to time; people tend to tuck themselves away when they are unhappy. Those negative feelings and behaviors can also be flags of distress, signaling "help me" while simultaneously pushing away the very people who care about you.
- **Premature aging.** Discontent and unhappiness show up on the body. Unhappy people slump more; they seem to have more wrinkle lines, from frowning so much; they may neglect their appearance, so hair, teeth, nails, and clothes look tired.

## The power of a smile

The good news is that you don't have to be happy to become happy. The moment you begin to smile, laugh, relax your shoulders, and wipe away the furrowed brow, two interesting things happen:

- The brain responds by releasing endorphins, which are the attraction hormones, and oxytocin—the "cuddle" hormone—making you feel instantly more positive, relaxed, and attractive.
- Those around you will behave more positively.

The result is that the brain learns to become happy, even if you didn't feel that way to begin with. The other secrets of happiness can be easily learned, too. Practicing them over time will see you through tougher times and carry others with you.

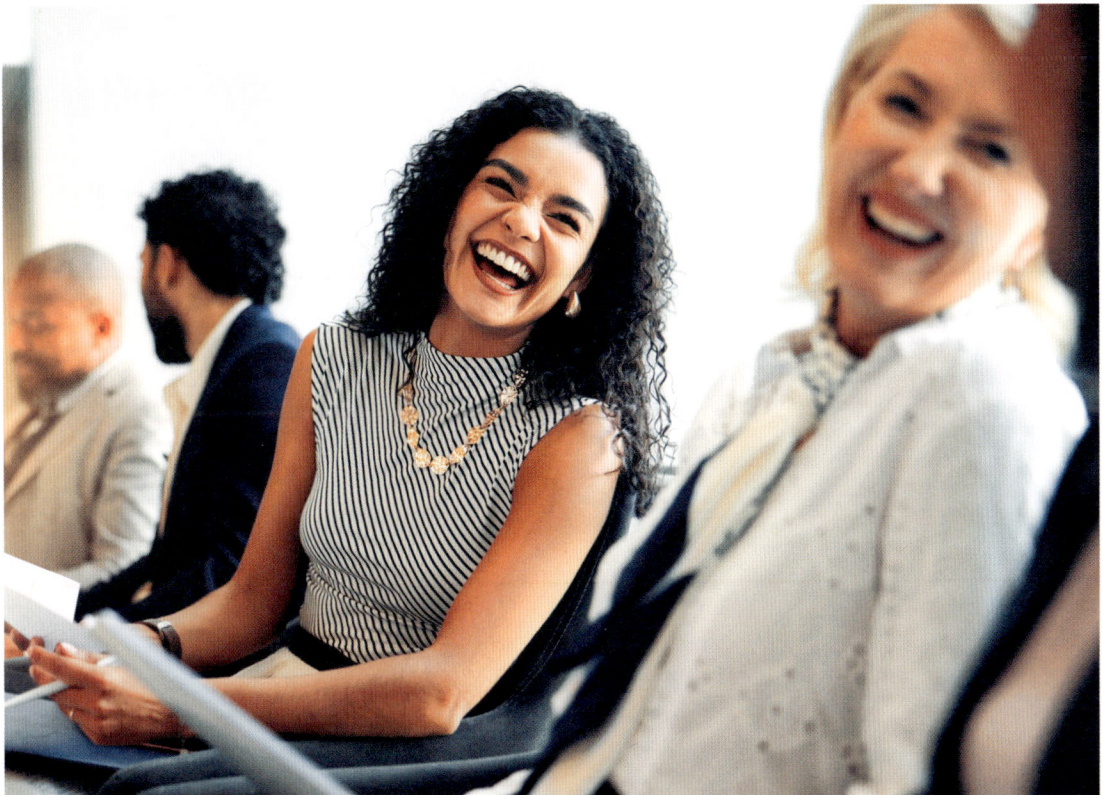

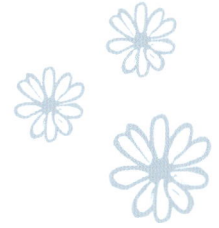

# Connect through empathy

Empathy is the capacity to understand the world from another's point of view. It is not about feeling sorry for someone or judging them; it is the ability to realize, "I have my opinion, but I can appreciate why you might see the situation differently."

Seeing the world through another's eyes lies at the heart of our capacity for kindness, community, kinship, and ultimately, happiness. Unless we can feel compassion for other people's troubles, unless we can try to appreciate what it must feel like to see things from other perspectives, we are simply islands—separated from one another by our indifference and selfishness.

Empathy is quite a sophisticated skill. We are not born with it. The frontal lobes of the brain are the area that helps us to develop reasoning skills, take responsibility, and apply our intelligence. They begin to develop at about two years old, which is also when we start to understand that not everyone sees the world the same way we do. The brain develops the capacity for empathy over time as we learn to share, take turns, forgive, and appreciate each other's differences. Empathy turns our focus outward instead of inward and helps us to be more understanding.

Why does empathy help us to find happiness? When we tune into other people's moods, we pick up on them, and they affect our own sense of wellbeing. Just as we can be affected by someone else's sadness, so too we can pick up on his or her feelings of happiness. When we are able to make other people feel happy, some of it rubs off on us. That explains why we tend to enjoy the company of upbeat, happy people.

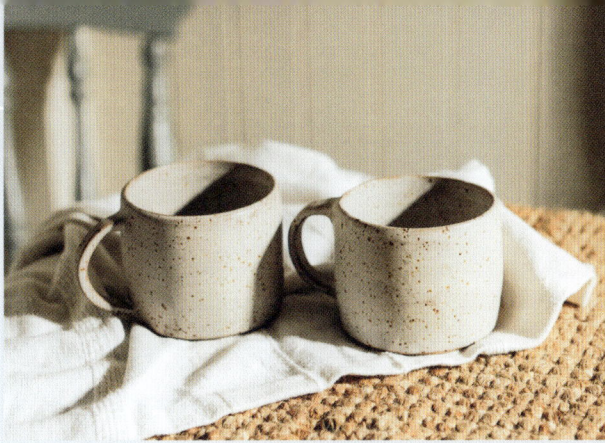

## PUT YOURSELF IN OTHERS' SHOES

Simple shifts in mindset can help you develop empathy and manage difficult situations better.

- **Suspend judgment.** Is there someone in your work or social life whose attitude drives you crazy? Does someone close to you irritate you with some of their habits and points of view? Try to suspend your judgment of them for a while and put yourself in their shoes. Why do you think they feel the need to be this way? Is it simply a defense mechanism? What does your irritation say about you? Is there something that you need to change?

- **Lighten up your language.** Who do you know who makes others feel happy to be around them? Listen to their choice of language; hear how they talk to other people. Are they using a lot of humor? Do they tend to frame things in a positive way and give credit where credit is due?

- **Look forward with hindsight.** There are times when being empathetic is challenging. If another driver were to run into your car, it might be hard to choose to see things from their point of view, but getting into a battle of words wouldn't resolve the situation any more quickly. In fact, it may make it worse. Try to look forward to a point where you can forgive their misjudgment; try to use empathy to let go of your anger, so that even if the car was badly damaged, the lasting impact would be on the vehicle, not on you.

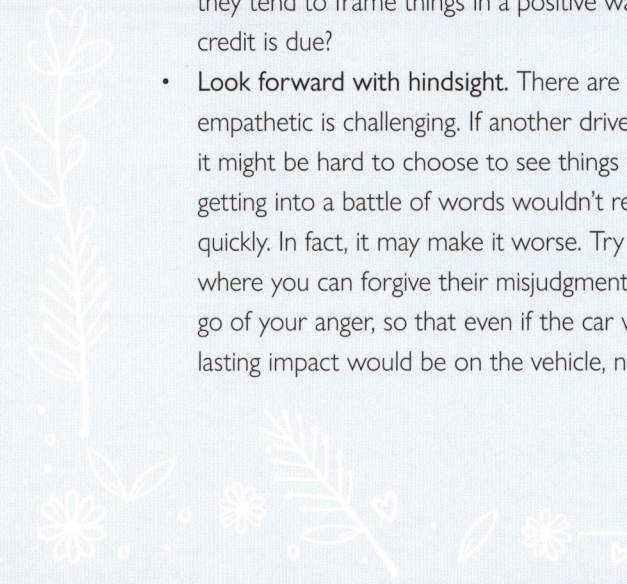

# Appreciate what you have

Many of us don't realize how happy we are because we take our current life so much for granted. We are always looking for faults and wishing for something else. Familiarity and routine threaten the specialness of what we have right now.

Most children and teenagers are blissfully complacent, especially those who have grown up with the material comforts of the western world. They take their education for granted; they expect to be fed; most will know that they are loved; and many will have clothes, gadgets, or vacations paid for by those who care for them. Of course, children deserve to feel secure and safe until they are ready to make their own way in the world. Very often it is not until children have left home for the first time, or started families themselves, that their sense of appreciation really begins.

However, if the pattern continues through life—getting without giving, receiving without reciprocation—neither the giver not the receiver benefit. Complacency shows up in a lack of awareness of others and an absence of gratitude. In the long-term, those who are complacent about their friendships, relationships, or material comforts without safeguarding them may lose them altogether.

Instead, let those who are close to you know how much you value them. Take note of what you have—your health, your home. Even a sunny day or a delicious meal are gifts to be grateful for.

Those who have had a difficult life still need to be alert to complacency. Being aware of what it feels like to be neglected or overlooked can help us to appreciate the value of care and kindness, and encourage us not to be complacent in learning how to treat others better than we are treated ourselves.

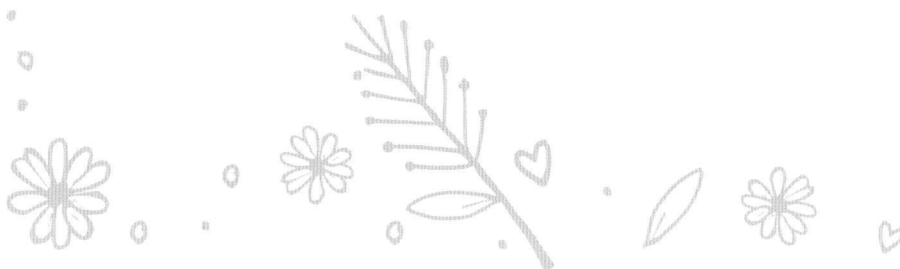

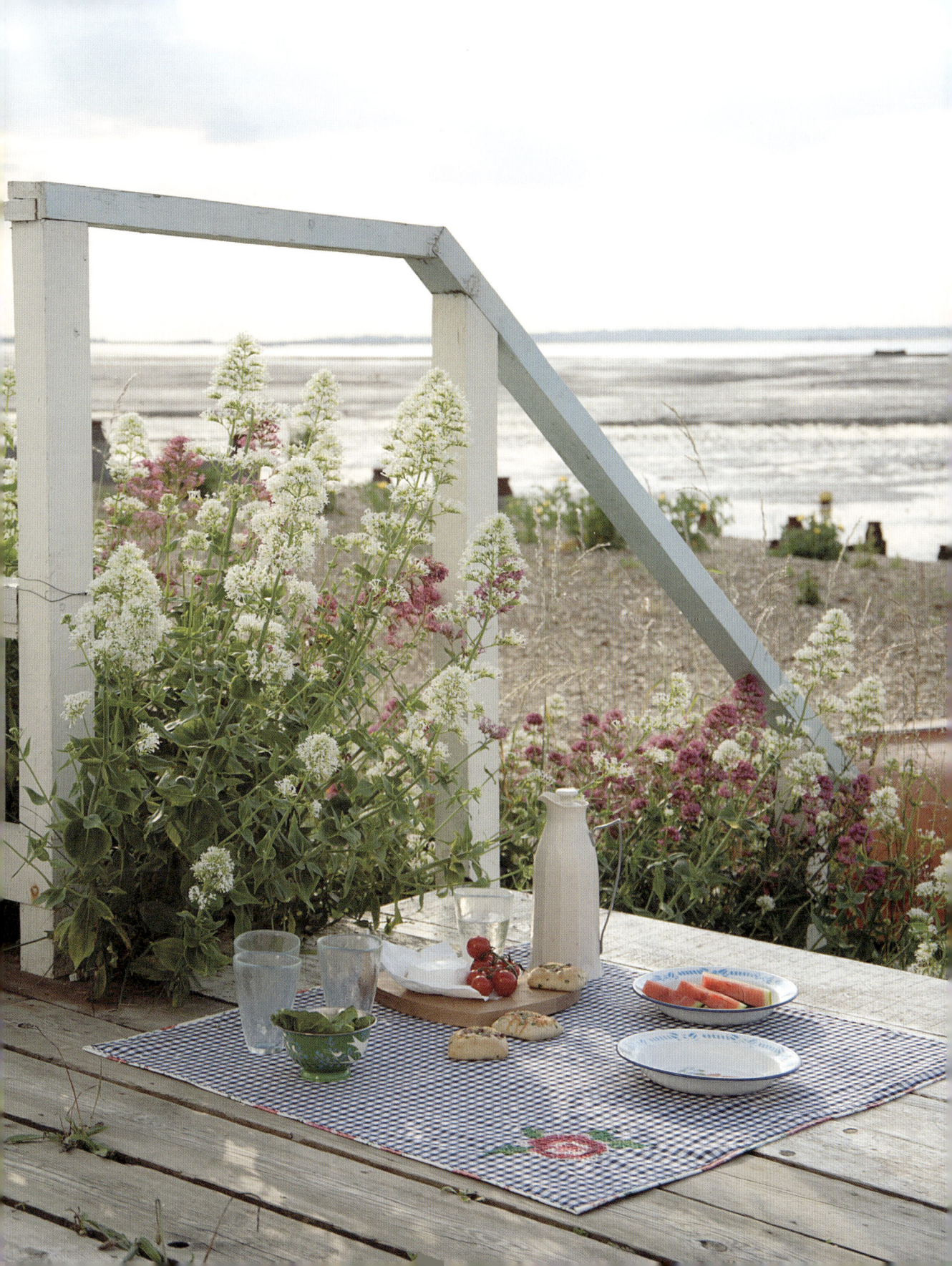

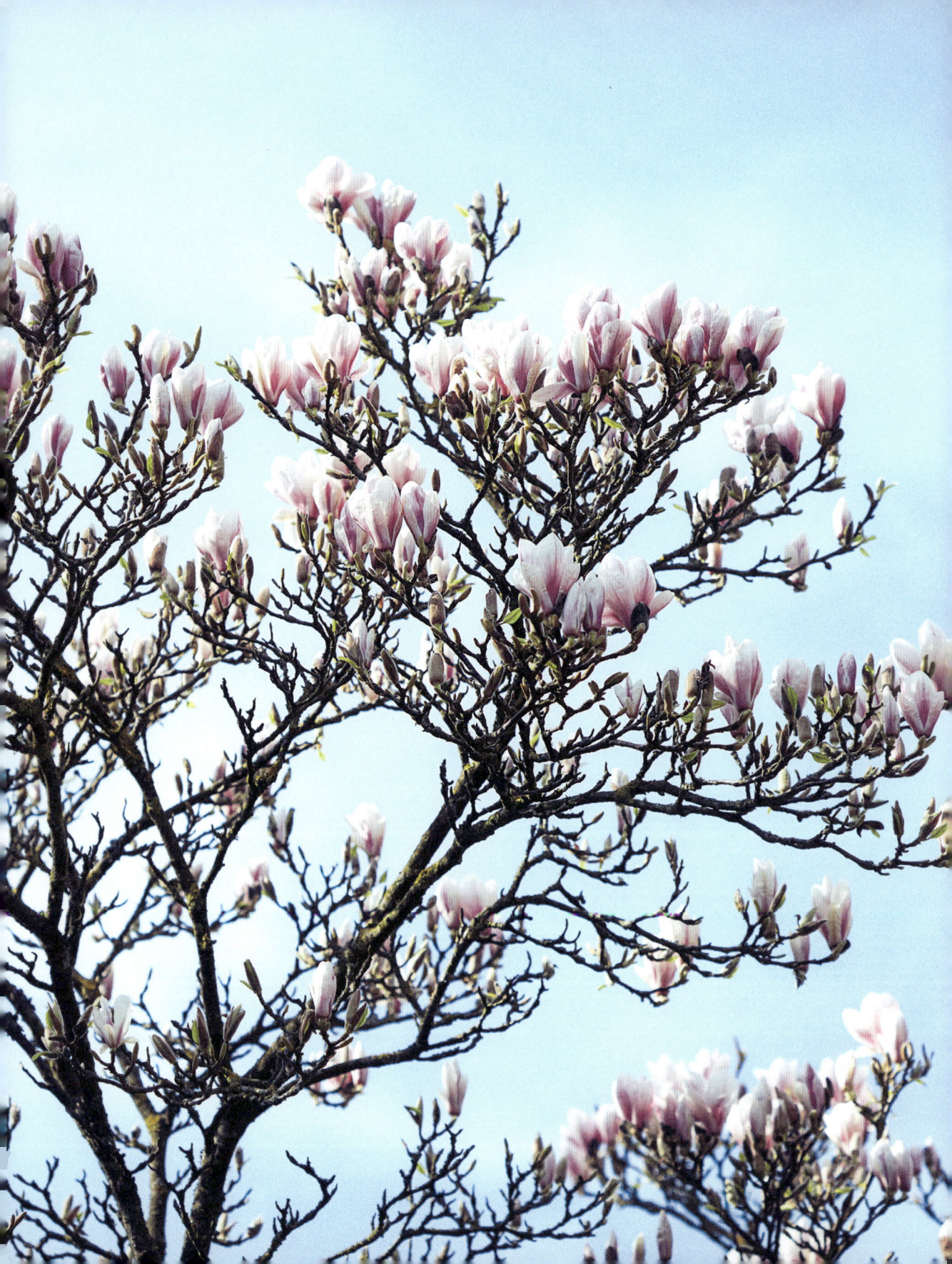

# BLESSING OF GRATITUDE

The blessing below has been inspired by Jack Kornfield, who is known around the world as a Buddhist practitioner and teacher. His many books are highly respected and his website is a rich source of ideas for meditation practice. His work consistently explains the rich value that such practice offers us in developing a more open-hearted, joyful, and grateful approach to life.

Let yourself sit quietly and in a relaxed fashion. Take a deep breath and then let go. Let your heart feel easy. Listen to your breath as you breathe in and out quietly and naturally. Allow your body to let go of all tension and become ready to receive this blessing:

*I offer my gratitude to the universe and all that is in it, for...*
*the friends I have been given;*
*the family I have been given;*
*the joy of life that I have been given;*
*the state of health and wellbeing that I have been given;*
*the neighbors that I have been given;*
*the teachers that I have been given;*
*the wisdom that I have been given;*
*the beauty of this earth, and the animals and birds that we have all been given;*
*my life and all that I have been given.*

Now continue to breathe in and out gently. Picture someone you care about, and think about them as they go about their daily life—and about the happiness and success you wish for them. With each breath, offer them your thanks from the bottom of your heart:

*May you always have joy in your heart.*
*May you always enjoy good fortune.*
*May your happiness continue to increase.*
*May you always have peace and wellbeing on this earth.*

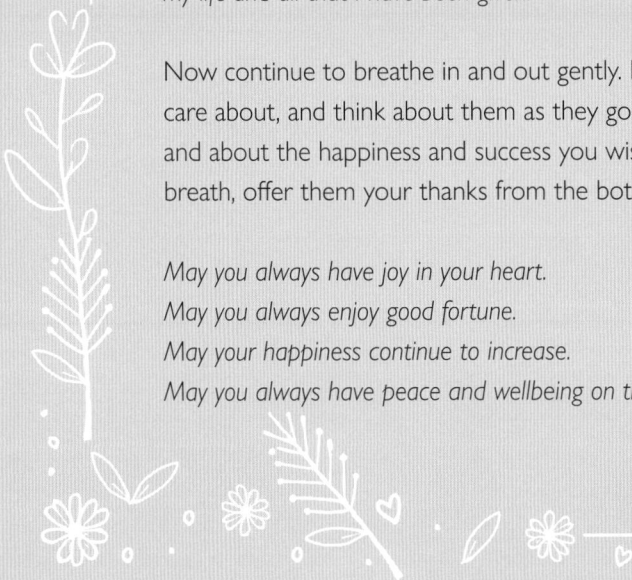

# The gift of giving

There is a secret to giving that not everyone has discovered but which is a source of optimism for the world. The good news is that giving to others is good for you. It will make you happy. It will make you feel better about yourself.

In 2010, the Charities Aid Foundation (CAF) joined with *The Sunday Times* to ask 69 of the UK's wealthiest people about the reasons for their philanthropy. The majority said the main reason was that they enjoyed giving. Over half wanted to leave a positive legacy. In the United States, Bill Gates is leading the way via the Bill and Melinda Gates Foundation. He has personally donated millions of dollars, and, with Warren Buffett, has launched The Giving Pledge, inviting billionaires to make a moral pledge to leave at least 50 percent of their fortunes as a legacy to philanthropic causes. Media mogul Simon Cowell has been quoted in the past as crediting Oprah Winfrey for helping him to discover how good it makes you feel to give money away as well as make it.

However, giving isn't just about money. The most valuable gift of all is your personal time—time spent in the service of others, listening and paying attention. The concept of service may seem old-fashioned in the modern world, but the nature of service goes much deeper than the odd good deed. When we are able to serve others, modestly, but putting the needs of the ego to one side, we become more humble, less focused on self, and more aware of the strengths of those around us.

Consider pledging to yourself today that you will consciously do one good deed per day, no matter how small, for the next ten days; and that, at the end of those ten days, you will repeat the pledge. Perhaps you'll make time for a coffee with a friend, pick up litter when see it, smile at a stranger... the possibilities are endless.

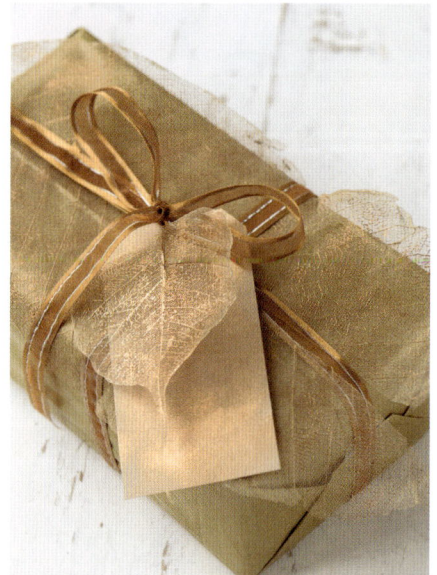

## SIMPLE WAYS TO CREATE A PERSONAL GIFT

Giving a gift is a special way to show gratitude, and need not be expensive. Choosing something with wit, care, originality, or attention to detail has far more value than a luxury label.

- Take a special photograph, and get family, friends, or colleagues to sign the mount. It will immediately become precious, even before you put it in a frame.

- Buy real ribbon made of natural fiber to tie up your parcels. It often costs no more than synthetic ribbon, and it makes your gift look extra-special. If possible, deliver the packages in person.

- Pass on a favorite book. It will mean even more to the recipient to know that it was yours and that you loved it.

- Bake! Homemade cookies or cake are always welcome, even if you are not a confident baker.

- Create a simple posy of handpicked home-grown or wild flowers, grasses, or leaves (just make sure you have permission to take them).

- Give something away. Most of us own far more than we need. As adults we may be hanging on to items that were precious to us in younger years—clothes or toys or paraphernalia from long-lost hobbies—but that someone else could be gaining pleasure from now. Giving things away is enormously liberating, especially when you know that objects from your past are adding joy to someone's present.

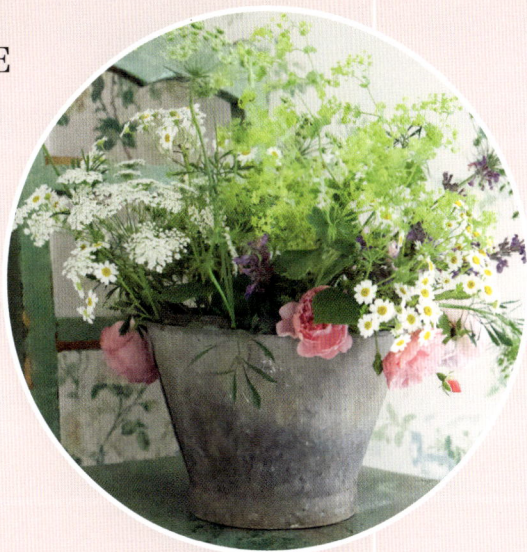

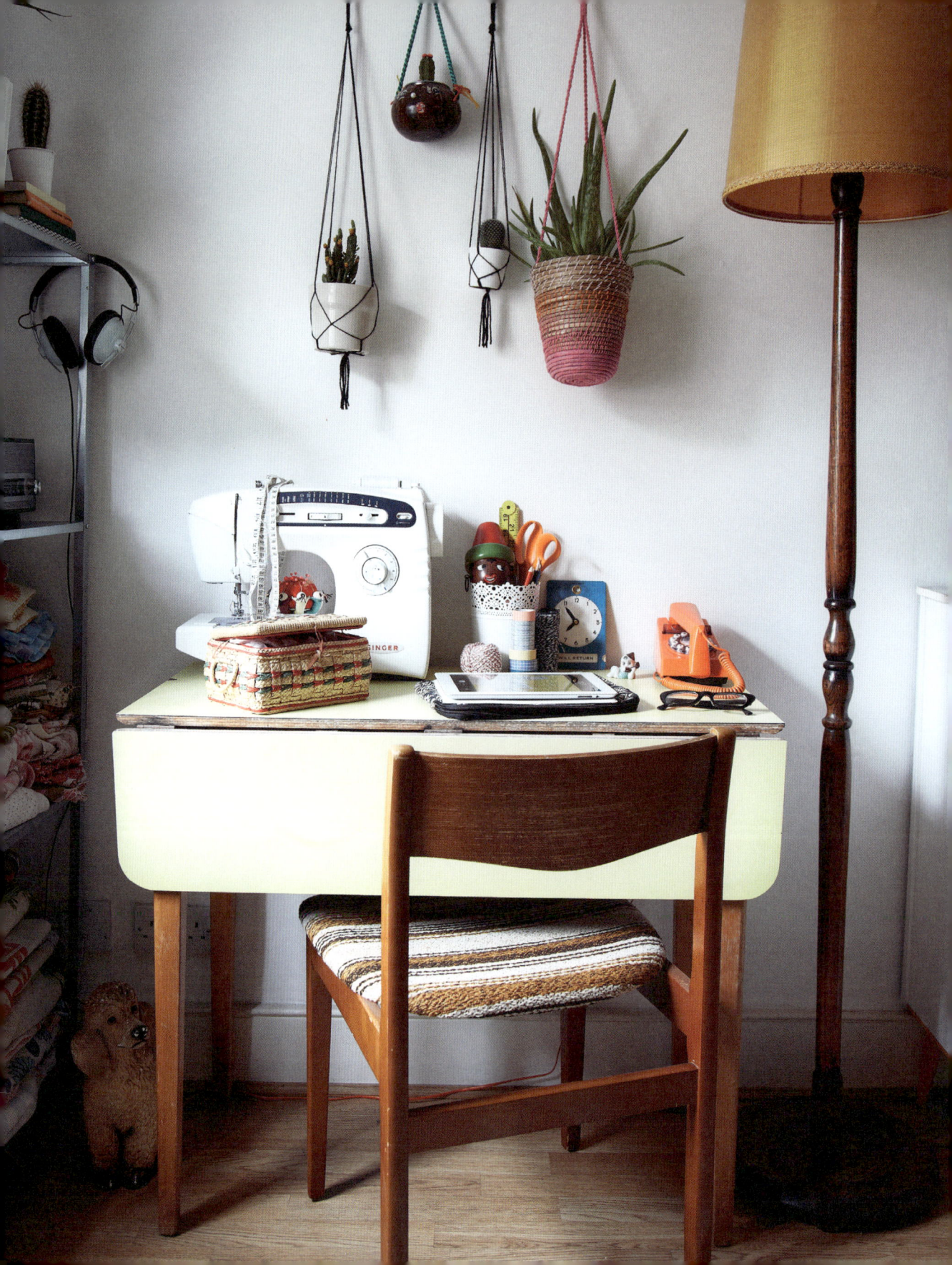

# Embrace your uniqueness

Everything you need to be happy lies within you right now. Wishing you were someone else with other talents and skills, or regretting that you did or didn't make a certain decision, will take you farther away from happiness.

Just consider the athletes in the Paralympics. They overcome a range of physical and mental challenges to come together from all over the world and compete with others who are the best in the world. The Paralympics shows us all that disabilities that would challenge many to remain positive are no barrier to success—tenacity, focus, training, guts, and skill gave each person a unique opportunity to succeed.

At the University of Pennsylvania in the USA, leading psychologist Dr Martin Seligman and colleagues are compiling an ongoing study into the factors that create authentic happiness. They found that one of the most important conditions of happiness is having strong awareness and appreciation of our own talents. Do you love to craft, sing, bake, or garden? When we understand what we are good at, we become more confident in our competence, and happier in ourselves. Looking yourself in the eye and appreciating who you are with all your beauty, skills, and potential, will take you to wherever you have the determination to be.

Appreciating your uniqueness requires you to pay as much attention to yourself as you would to other people; it means listening to the complimentary things that people might say and believing that there is merit in them. It also means absorbing criticism, no matter how hard it is to hear, and realizing that there are things about yourself that you might choose to improve or change.

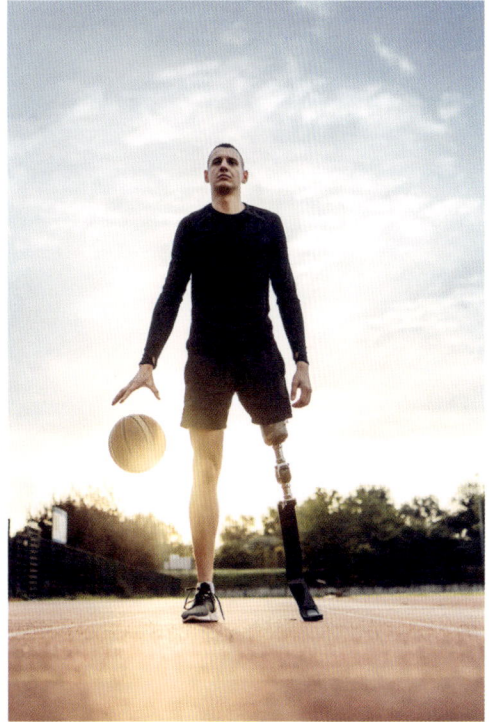

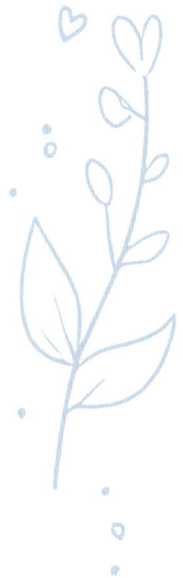

# Take risks

For most of our lives, we may choose to live within a personal comfort zone of familiarity and safety; in doing so we think we remain safe from harm and away from failure. But the truth is that the safer we feel, the more afraid we become, because doing something unfamiliar feels increasingly daunting.

Have you the courage to let go of the person you think you are right now in order to find happiness? Are you brave enough to live life to the full? A very safe life can become an anxious life, lived within self-limiting boundaries. Happiness may become unhappiness because we are not living a life that is fulfilled. Interestingly, it is when we risk failure that we learn the most; and it is when we start to stretch ourselves that our potential for happiness increases.

What is your attitude to new situations? Do you embrace them fully and worry about the consequences afterward; or do you choose not to try because you don't want to risk failure? Whatever your attitude, decide on a new challenge and choose to behave in a way that is opposite to your usual behavior. If you are risk-averse, just say yes to the opportunity; if you usually leap before thinking, decide this time to ask advice or create a plan. The new risk-taker may discover that they are better at thinking on their feet than they realized; the new planner may discover that when fully prepared, they can achieve even greater heights.

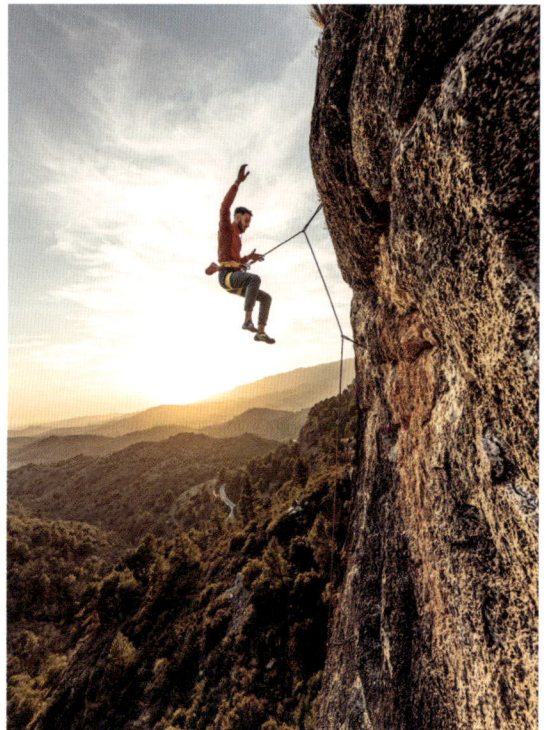

## REDEFINING WHO YOU ARE

Consider the following:

- What role do you play? Sometimes we are so attached to a particular view of ourselves that we don't realize that it is holding us back.
- What words do you use to describe yourself? Are you the shy one, the sporty one, the clever one, the one who is hopeless at x, y, or z?
- Where do the origins of those beliefs come from? Are they really true?
- What opportunities are you not taking because you can't see yourself in the role?

By changing how we think of ourselves, we can become more open to what life has to offer. The brain appreciates clear direction and will fulfill instructions if you keep them repeating them over a period time. Try telling yourself some different labels, such as:

- I have courage
- I have talent
- I have the tenacity to succeed
- I am a dancer
- I am a singer
- I am good at sport
- I am an attractive person
- I am sociable
- I am happy

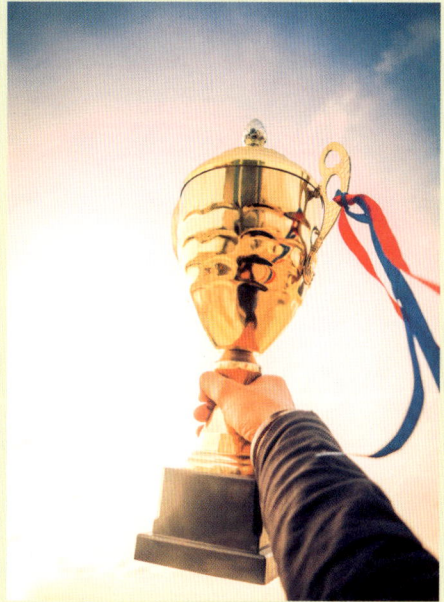

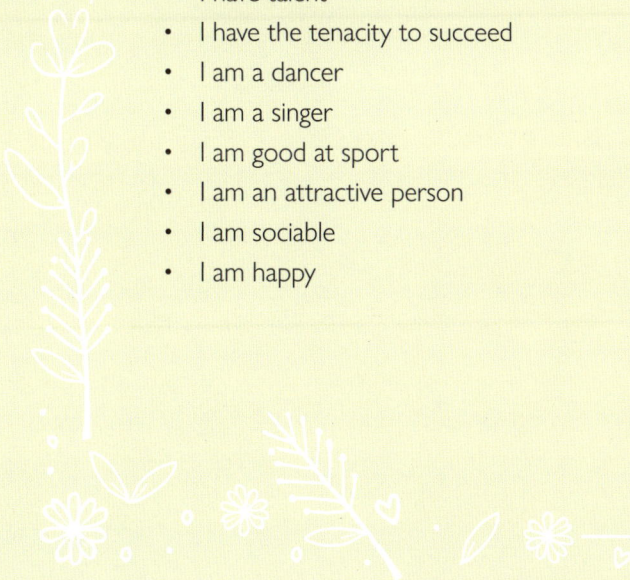

# Practice calm for more peace

Finding a place to be still and calm is wonderfully relaxing. Finding your way to a place of calm inside your mind, is to find a place where transformation can occur and peace can be found.

This is the role of prayer and meditation and much of the function of spiritual rituals. The aim is to change your state of mind from a place of busy-ness to one of stillness and contemplation. Some people find a more active route to calm, via yoga, tai chi, chanting, or running; others find it by walking through the countryside or city in the cool of the morning. However you get there, we all need periods of calm and quiet order. In those moments when we are simply still, transition takes place and things become clearer in our minds.

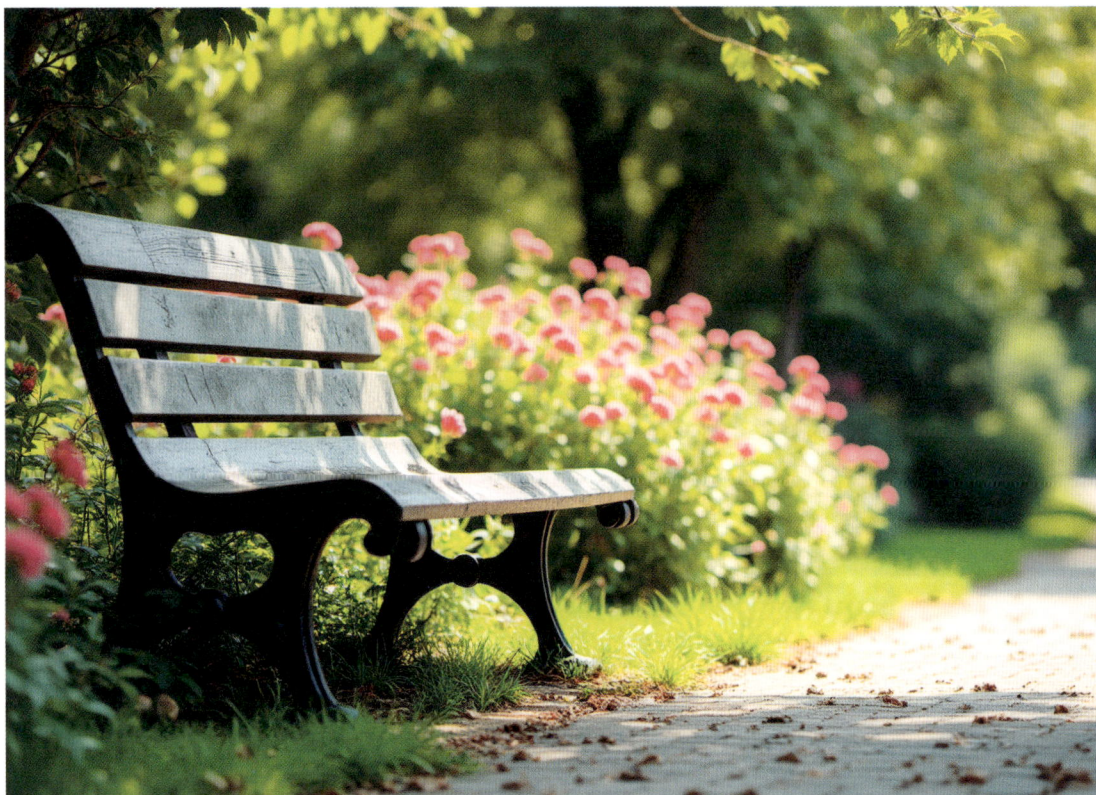

## JUST BREATHE

At its simplest level, finding a route to calm is about breathing. Choose a place where there is no likelihood of interruption or distractions and that is neither too hot nor too cold.

- Lie down on your back on the floor.
- Let your feet flop outward and relax your hands so that your palms, facing up, and fingers find their own natural position.
- Close your eyes and relax your mind.
- Don't worry about where your thoughts are taking you. Don't focus on them. Just let them come and go as they please.
- Focus on your breath.
- Breathe in deeply; and then breathe out fully; breathe in fully and breathe out fully.
- Let your breath find its own rhythm, but keep the breaths deep.
- Maintain this for as long as you feel comfortable.
- Focus only on your breath.

You may find that when you first try to do this, you fall asleep. You may find, too, that your breath is coming from your upper body instead of your lower diaphragm and that you are holding your breath instead of letting it flow. Try to practice breathing with your hand on your belly. It should inflate with the in-breath and deflate with the out-breath. It will come with practice.

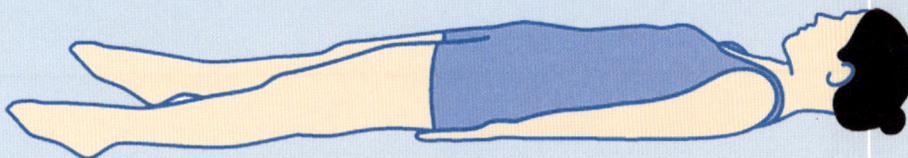

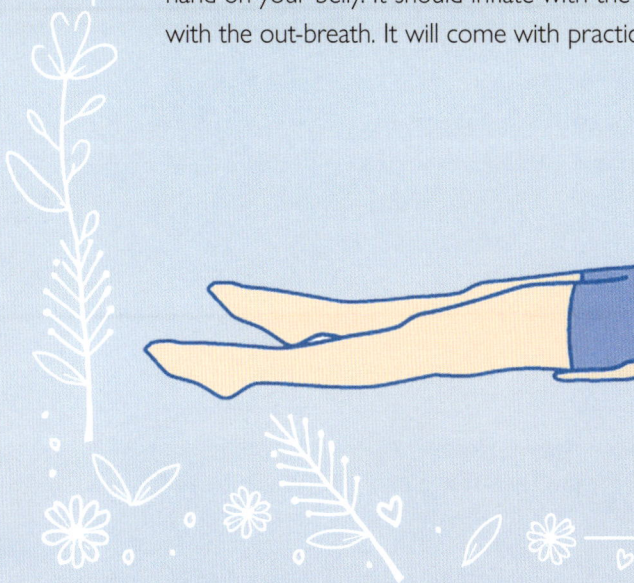

# Enjoy your journey

When we look back over the course of life, it will not be the detail of the profit and loss sheet, the pressure of deadlines, or the escalating cost of groceries that you will remember—it will be the great times with friends, the joy of watching your children in the school play, a special day in a beautiful location, the pleasure of walking your dog, the first time you heard your favorite piece of music, shared moments with loved ones.

Omar Havana is an international photojournalist with a social conscience. His striking images do more for human rights than speeches and editorial could ever do alone. His series of images of families scratching a living in a vast Cambodian landfill site have been seen by millions around the world. Among these, one picture in particular stands out. A young girl, aged about four, stands alone in the middle of an endless ocean of debris. With a tatty sack in her hands, she looks directly at his camera and smiles, her face lit up in joy. Was it the novelty of being noticed, and having her photo taken? Partly, perhaps. But what touches your heart when looking at his picture is the sense that this little girl, who knows no way of life other than dire poverty, seems rich in her soul—because she knows how to be happy.

For those of us who have the opportunity to choose our journey in life, such an image is a real wake-up call. Who are we to feel less than satisfied with life when others need so much and yet find contentment in what they've got?

Children in general seem preprogramed for happiness. They have the power of imagination to help if something happens to ruin their day. Children often talk in superlatives—and they really notice the details. When something is in favor, it is immediately "best" or "favorite" and essential to life (although things may fall out of favor just as quickly). Can you still remember your favorite childhood toy, picture book, or TV show? That part of your journey is etched in your memory forever.

As adults, we tend to swap play and imagination for the routine of work and a busy diary. The nine-to-five all too often becomes a means to an end rather than a conscious journey. We no longer pay attention to the details and don't always fully absorb the joy that our journey is giving us. Our challenge is to spend less time focused solely on the task or the rewards, and more on noticing the happiness to be had in the present moment.

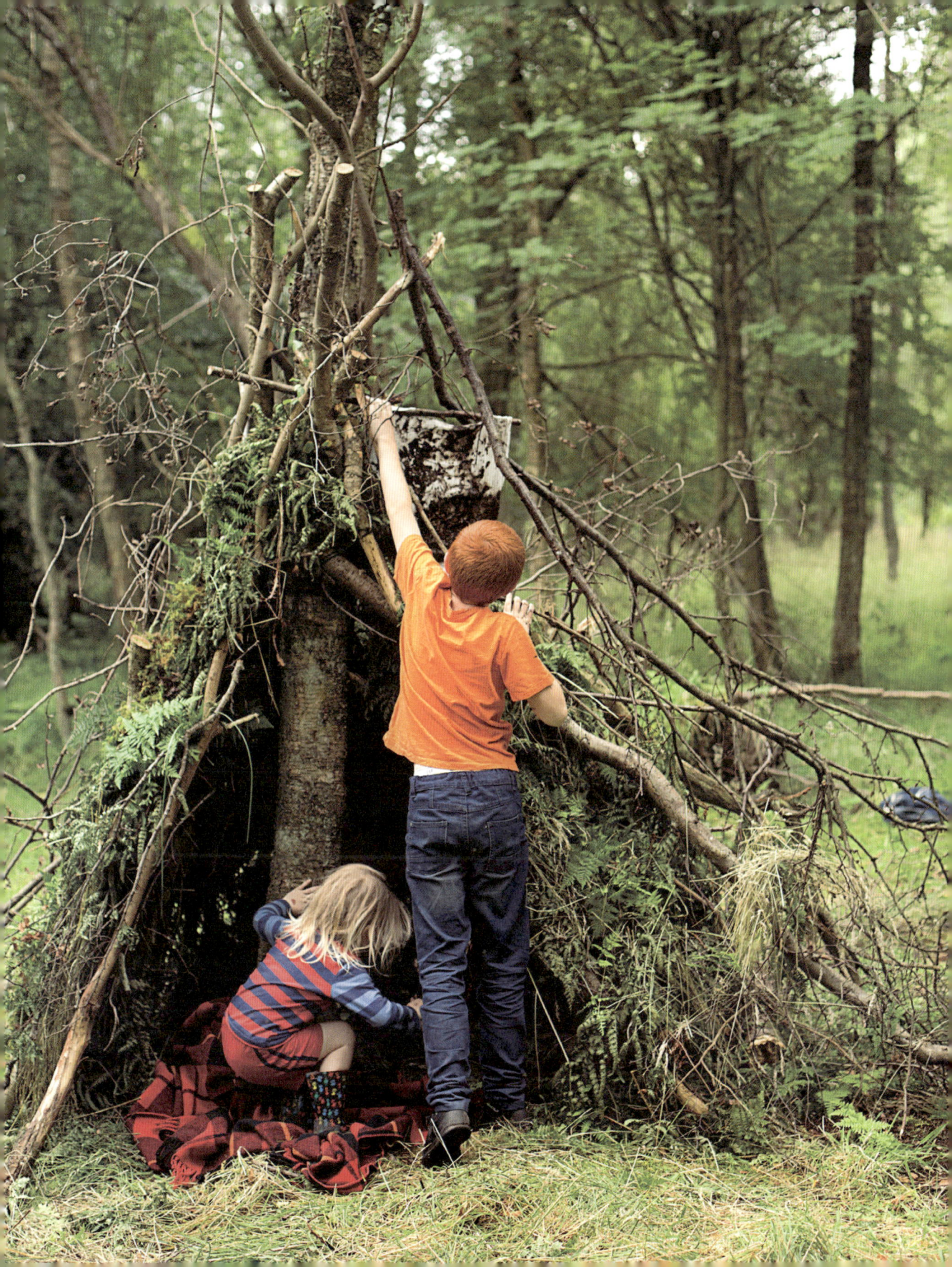

## KEEP A HAPPINESS JOURNAL

Writers and artists will often keep notebooks or draw sketches of things that have caught their attention. You, too, can keep journal as a place to capture memories of the past and record each day's events that gave you pause for thought.

The inner journey that we travel in life has the potential to be endlessly rich and varied; it provides opportunities to explore and develop our true selves in a way that can open up our minds to new opportunities of who we are and what we might be. The various forms of social media have their role to play, but sometimes, when we share our thoughts with the world, we offer the edited version. We present ourselves as we would like to be seen, rather than revealing what we really feel.

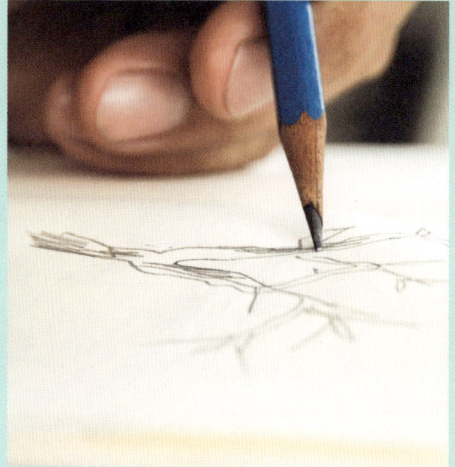

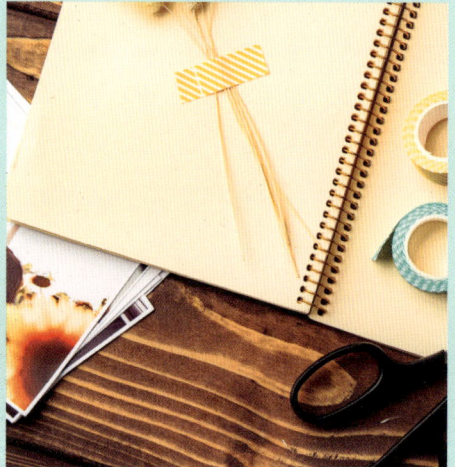

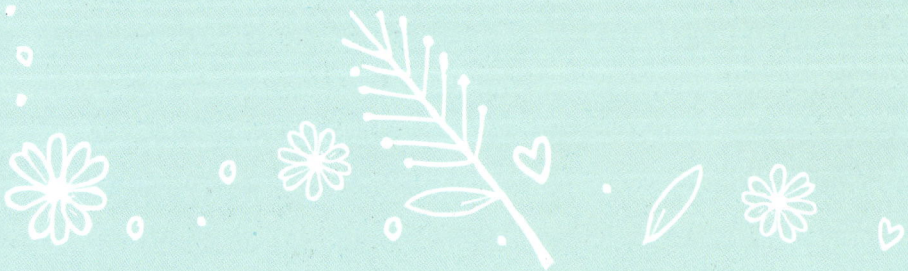

Deciding to keep a happiness journal can be a wonderful way of tuning in to the here and now and reminding yourself to pay attention to the present. Getting into the habit of writing down, photographing, painting, or capturing in some way those moments when you have felt alive, content, or joyful has several benefits:

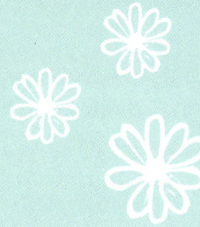

- You will immediately feel the experience more intensely, as you seek to capture it.
- Your happiness radar will increase its powers of detection. The more you look, the more you will see reasons to be happy.
- It will serve as a record of happy moments and as a pick-me-up for those times when you feel blue.
- It will encourage you to think beyond the experience of the moment, to make connections between different experiences, and to learn more about yourself.

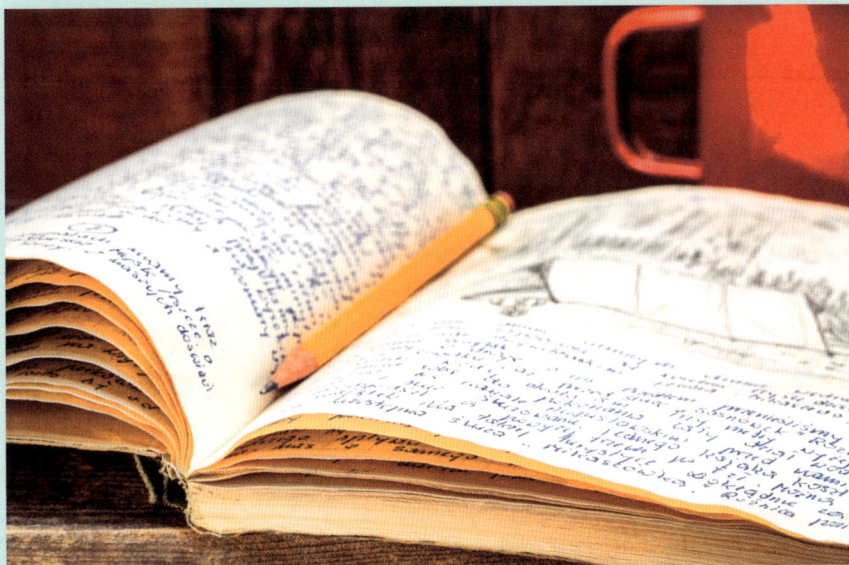

# Helpful reminders

Your future happiness begins in the present moment. Yesterday has gone; nothing you do or say can change the past—but tomorrow and the days ahead are unchartered territory. There is so much you can do to influence the way your future evolves and what you feel about it.

Living life consciously puts more emphasis on the present moment. It brings our present actions into clear focus, encouraging us to mind what we think and to think about what we do and say. Paying attention to the present moment nurtures careful observation and appreciation of the things around us; it puts us in closer touch with our feelings, our reactions, and our intuition, because there are no distractions.

Here are a few instant mood switchers that can be used when groans and grumbles threaten to chase away the chance of happiness on a daily basis. Life often presents moments of frustration, stress, or sadness, and it's during these times that having simple, effective tools to shift your mindset can make a big difference. These behaviors are easy to implement and are designed to help you regain a sense of balance and positivity, even in the midst of everyday challenges.

## Breathe consciously and stand up straight

The body holds tension. When we feel anxious, our breathing becomes shallow and our shoulders rise. By taking deep breaths and shaking out the shoulders, you will release tension, improve your posture, and immediately feel lighter and happier.

## Look after your body

Make time to have a soak in the bath, or a steaming power shower; keep your hair trimmed; wear your favorite shirt; massage your skin. The skin is the largest organ of the body. It needs oxygen and nutrients to keep healthy and keep you protected. If you feel good physically, you will feel better mentally. Get enough sleep. It is hard to feel happy if you are exhausted.
(See also Chapter 3.)

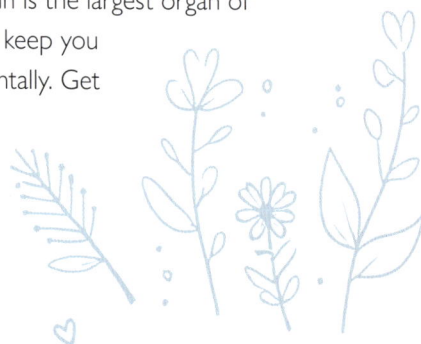

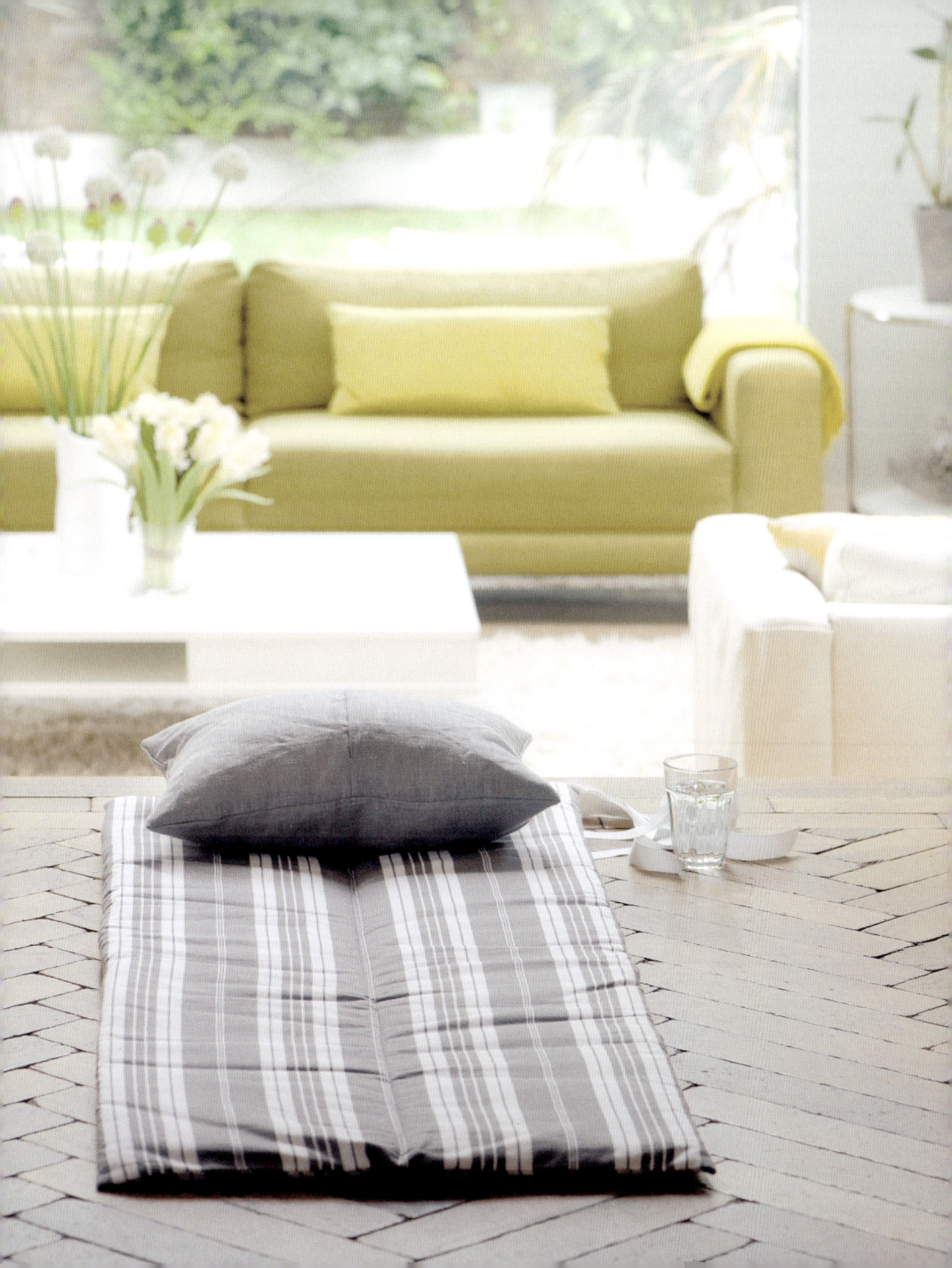

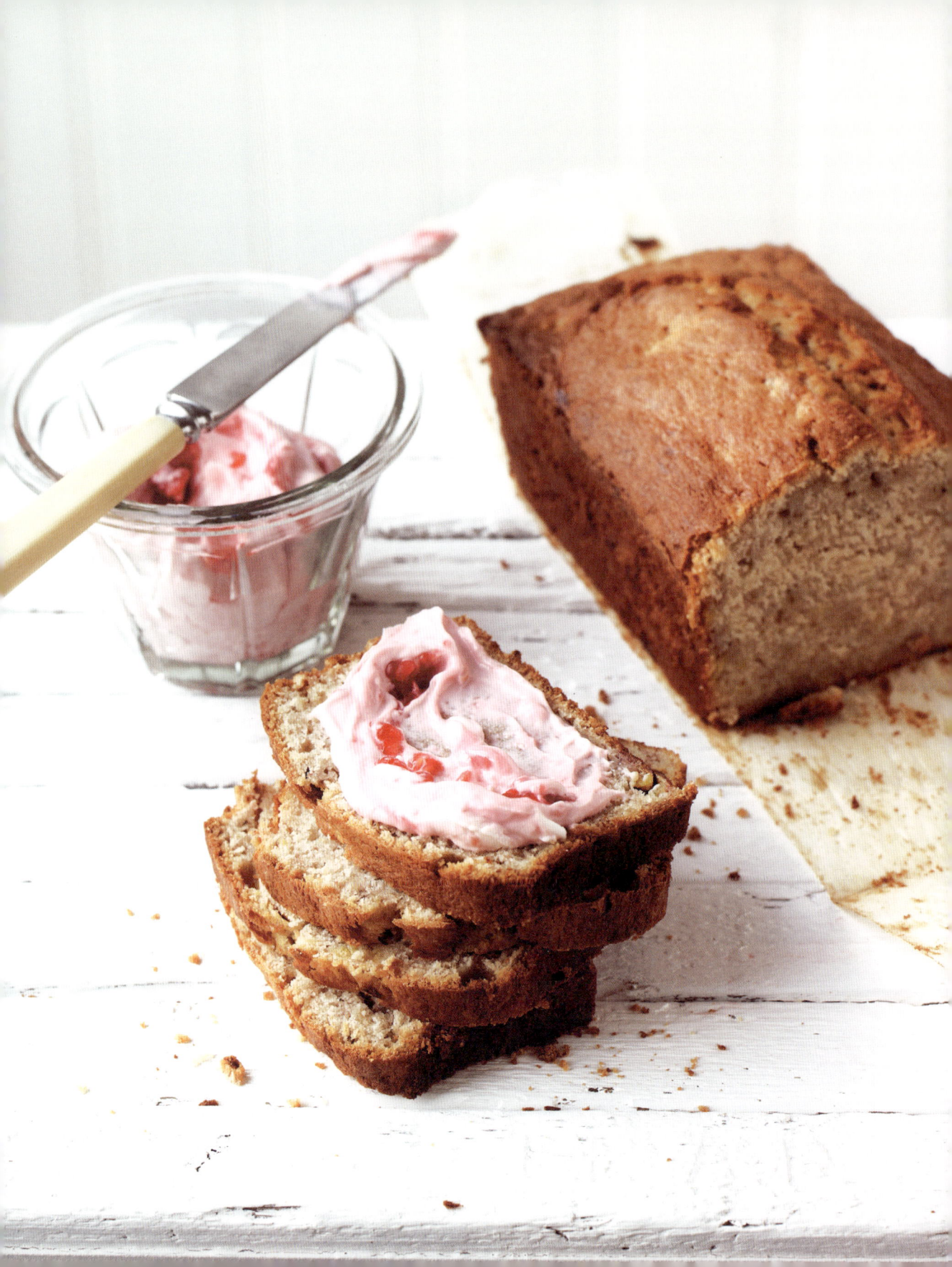

## Awaken your senses

Your senses send messages to the brain. When your senses are alert, you feel more alive. Focus fully on what you are doing at every moment of the day. There is joy to be had in every task: the sight of a robin hopping about while you are weeding; the smell of the ingredients while you are baking; the sound of your children chattering while discovering their world; the hug or touch of a friend or lover. Appreciating the small things awakens awareness of the bigger things, and helps to put us back in touch with our true selves.

## Watch your language

The moment you hear yourself think or say passive words, such as "I wish/should/might/can't," swap them for more active words, such as "I can," "I will," or "I am." You will feel instantly happier if your choice of language puts you in control of your life.

## Learn to say no

Busy people tend to say yes to things because they can. Unassertive people tend to say yes to things because they can't quite manage to say no. A simple sentence, such as, "I won't be able to do that for you because I am already very busy/fully committed/doing something else," will get you out of trouble.

## Laugh

Laughter wipes away tension in a single breath and turns a frowning face into one that is alive and beautiful. It doesn't take much to trigger a giggle: just thinking about something funny that has happened in the past can provoke laughter and increase joy. Phone a friend, tell a silly joke, read a favorite cartoon strip, look for the absurd in every situation. Laugh—several times a day.

## Be kind to others

Studies have proven again and again that the quickest and most satisfying route to finding happiness is not to think about yourself all the time, but to focus on other people and what they need instead. As human beings, we are social creatures who like to be connected to one another. Giving and gratitude are essential ingredients in the formulation and experience of happiness.

## Listen

When we tune in to what people are really saying, we feel more strongly connected to them and more compassionate. When we feel heard and understood we feel more loved, better supported, more contented, and we are more likely to listen to and help others.

# RESOURCES

## CBD AND ESSENTIAL OILS LEARNING RESOURCES

www.aromatics.com/pages/learning-guides
www.projectcbd.org

## CBD SOURCES

www.rosebudcbd.com (US)
www.shop-poplar.com (US/UK/EU/CA/ROW)
www.charlottesweb.com (US)
www.blacktiecbd.net (US)
www.love-hemp.com (UK/EU)
www.cbd-guru.co.uk (UK/EU/ROW)

## ESSENTIAL OILS SOURCES

www.aromatics.com (US/UK/EU/CA/ROW)
www.oshadhi.co.uk (UK/EU)
www.newdirectionsaromatics.ca (US/CA)
www.escents.ca (US/CA)
www.edensgarden.com (US/UK/EU/CA/ROW)
www.baseformula.com (UK)
www.nealsyardremedies.com (UK/EU)

## FURTHER READING

Page 48: Melissa R. Marselle et al., "Moving beyond Green: Exploring the Relationship of Environment Type and Indicators of Perceived Environmental Quality on Emotional Well-Being following Group Walks," *International Journal of Environmental Research and Public Health*, 12/1 (2015), pp. 106–130.

Page 49: Gregory N. Bratman et al., "Nature Experience Reduces Rumination and Subgenual Prefrontal Cortex Activation," *Proceedings of the National Academy of Sciences of the United States of America*, 112/28 (July 14, 2015), www.pnas.org/content/112/28/8567

Page 51: Ahmad Hassan et al., "Effects of Walking in Bamboo Forest and City Environments on Brainwave Activity in Young Adults," *Evidence-based Complementary and Alternative Medicine*, 2018, www.hindawi.com/journals/cam/2018/9653857

Page 125: A more complete version of the meditation can be found at "Meditation on Gratitude and Joy." www.jackkornfield.com/meditation-gratitude-joy

# CREDITS

## TEXT CREDITS

© **Rika K. Keck:** pages 10–33, 36–37
© **Anna Black:** pages 34–35, 40–41, 44–45, 72–87
© **Noelle Renée Kovary:** pages 40–41, 44–47, 52–69
© **Lois Blyth:** pages 42–43, 108–141
© **Alice Peck:** pages 48–51
© **Colleen Quinn:** pages 88–105

## IMAGE CREDITS

Key: t = top, c = center, b = bottom, l = left, r = right

© **Ryland Peters and Small,** by the following photographers: **Caroline Arber:** pages 2, 123, 126, 139; **Ed Anderson:** pages 3, 8, 13, 16, 30; **Joanne Murphy:** pages 4, 89, 90, 97, 98, 101, 102, 104, 105; **Shirlie Kemp:** pages 5c, 127; **Edina van der Wyck:** pages 5r, 113; **Camila Gray:** page 11; **Mowie Kay:** pages 19, 22, 25, 28; **Stuart West:** pages 27, 29t, 33t, 106; **Susan Bell:** page 32b; **Simon Brown:** page 35; **Chris Everard:** page 41; **Georgia Glynn-Smith:** page 42; **Winfried Heinze:** page 43; **Penny Wincer:** pages 47, 87; **Mari Magnusson:** page 49; **Dylan Drummond and Terry Benson:** pages 50, 109, 135; **Steve Dew:** pages 55, 56, 57r, 63, 64b, 68; **Anthony Duke:** pages 60, 64t, 67, 133; **Debi Treloar:** page 70; **Andrew Wood:** page 73; **Catherine Gratwicke:** page 78; **Rachel Whiting:** page 81; **Claire Winfield:** page 93; **David Merewether:** page 115; **Becky Maynes:** page 117; **Kim Lightbody:** page 124; **Emma Mitchell and James Gardiner:** page 128; **Kate Whitaker:** page 140

© **Adobestock.com** and the following creators: **Anom S.:** floral art throughout; **Alex Pios:** pages 1, 132; **Monster Ztudio:** page 51, 83; **svsunny:** page 14; **Artem Shadrin:** pages 15t, 26; **Elenathewise:** page 15ct; **mizina:** page 15cb; **vm2002:** page 15b; **New Africa:** page 17t, 77, 96; **Subbotina Anna:** page 17ct; **IRINA:** page 17cb; **Elena Moiseeva:** page 17b; **Виктория Попова:** page 18; **Natalia:** page 21t; **Jiri Hera:** page 21bl; **nata_vkusidey:** page 21bc; **monticellllo:** page 21br; **Алина Битта:** page 29b; **vlaru:** page 32t; **al62:** page 32c; **manuta:** page 33b; **Vladislav Noseek:** page 36t; **noirchocolate:** page 36b; **Peter Hermes Furian:** page 37; **Creativa Images:** page 38; **Joie Digital Assets:** page 45; **Vulp:** page 48; **Svetlana Khutornaia:** page 52; **Cristina:** page 53; **kite_rin:** page 54; **AntonioDiaz:** page 57l; **junky_jess:** page 59; **fizkes:** page 61, 65; **Damir Khabirov:** page 62; **kegfire:** page 66; **undrey:** page 69; **oatawa:** page 74; **gpointstudio:** page 82; **Anastasiia:** page 84; **daffodilred:** page 95; **Ameer:** page 110; **flyalone:** page 112; **Mumtaaz Dharsey/peopleimages.com:** page 116t; **Marinela:** page 116b; **peopleimages.com:** page 119; **Reuben:** page 121; **Dusan Petkovic:** page 129; **VICTOR:** page 130; **35mm:** page 131; **ponsulak:** page 136t; **fotofabrika:** page 136b; **MarekPhotoDesign.com:** page 137

# INDEX